Reclaiming the Joy of a Church Vocation

THE WAY TO WELLNESS FOR THE NON-ORDAINED IN CHURCH AND SCHOOL MINISTRIES

Darrell W. Zimmerman

Grace Place Wellness Ministries

Reclaiming the Joy of a Church Vocation is a resource that every church worker should add to their professional library. Darrell Zimmerman shares his personal wellness journey with a solid foundation in God's Word and an honest assessment of the path to restoring joy in ministry. This inspirational resource can be used for personal study or with team members. What a blessing to all church workers serving in ministries in challenging times!

Dr. Rebecca Schmidt, Director of School Ministry, LCMS

Ministry in the church is such a beautiful vocation filled with a lot of joy but with it comes many challenges that can affect the health and wellness of the worker. So many resources focus on the wellness of the ordained pastor, but this book especially focuses on the non-ordained worker in the church and school, noting the unique differences and challenges that these workers face in ministry and in their personal lives. It is filled with real-life stories, scripture, thoughtful questions to consider, and much encouragement for the daily life of those who serve in the church. It's an opportunity to take a pause to read and reflect and become mindful of how you can seek ways to grow in your wellness to best serve the Kingdom. Highly recommended for the non-ordained worker (and maybe the pastor too!).

Dr. Debbie Arfsten, (DCE) Program Director, Concordia University Chicago

Reverend Zimmerman is perfectly accurate in his description of the ministry life of a Commissioned Church Worker in *Reclaiming the Joy of a Church Vocation*. His sensitivity to the stresses and dilemmas faced by congregational workers is realistic. His lessons are powerful. As a former Congregational Commissioned Worker and School Administrator, I believe that this book is a must in the professional development of a congregational worker. Faculties should adopt it as a basis for regular discussion at faculty meetings.

Dr. Joseph Bordeaux, Lutheran School Principal (ret.)

Reclaiming the Joy of a Church Vocation is such a timely read for ALL commissioned ministers. Following this read, I rediscovered how to assess a better plan for my own personal wellbeing. I am convinced that this book and its application will help church work professionals develop strategies where all members of a ministry team will flourish as Christ-like servant leaders in their homes, workplaces and in community. Darrell has refueled this worker for continued team ministry and service!

James Bradshaw
Assistant to the President, Education and Youth, Kansas District, LCMS

Having grown up as the child of two church workers, and joining the teaching ministry along with my husband, I have experienced first-hand both the joys and hardships of ministry. Darrell's book not only acknowledges the challenges faced for all people in ministry, but also recognizes the importance of "daily healing." I found Darrell's book to be a much-needed read after 20+ years of teaching. Knowing I probably have an equal number of years remaining in my career, it was an important refresh. This book allowed me to step back, reflect on where joy is present and where it is lacking, and examine how I can better equip myself with daily healing practices for my spiritual and physical health.

Erica Spangler, Parochial School Teacher

When ministers aren't ministering well, or being ministered to, where can they turn? Darrell Zimmerman's book, *Reclaiming the Joy of Ministry*, is a wonderful place to start. Pastor Zimmerman has a great capacity for being able to dwell as a faithful companion in the hard spaces that arise in any believer's life, but in this book, he gifts that ability to fellow church workers. The life of a pastor, deaconess, DCE or other called worker is often a strange mix of life in the spotlight and life pushed to the shadows. In his writing, Pastor Zimmerman gently leads church workers to hold up the different aspects of their lives to the Light of truth, looking for broken boundaries or warped responsibilities. With the guiding power of the Spirit, Darrell then helps church workers to accept healing and grace for themselves, and reestablish lives of joy in Christ.

Deaconess Kristina Paul, Salem Lutheran, Affton, MO

I really enjoyed reading this book. Darrell offers many practical thoughts and solutions to find joy in ministry. Reading the book was refreshing and a reminder to me of why I love doing what I do and what are some areas that I can work on to strengthen my joy in ministry.

Rehema Kavugha, DCE, Synod Relations Manager, Lutheran Church Extension Fund

Accolades for the precursor to this volume: *Reclaiming the Joy of Ministry: The Grace Place Way to Church Worker Wellness*

Darrell Zimmerman has written a wonderful book full of wisdom and spiritual truth. Using the stories of the prophet Elijah as both a mirror and window into Christian ministry, Darrell combines rich theological insight, intimate personal experience and wise counsel to create a book that will penetrate to the heart of ministers and their spouses. More than once I saw myself—and my inner life—revealed in these pages. But more than that, Reclaiming the Joy of Ministry never left me in the dark wondering, "What do I do now?" Rather, Zimmerman encourages, leads, comforts and provides greatly needed help. *Reclaiming the Joy of Ministry* is a spiritually strengthening journey that richly rewards anyone who makes the trip.

Dr. Timothy E. Saleska, Dean of Ministerial Formation, Concordia Seminary, St. Louis

This is a very practical guide for anyone looking to reclaim the joy of ministry. Joy fuels ministry! Darrell Zimmerman and Grace Place Wellness Ministries have provided some honest, challenging and fruitful lessons for those who have lost their joy in ministry to journey towards a more resilient and healthy service in relationship to God and to their neighbor. Recognizing that "You can't preach what you don't know" we are reminded that Jesus doesn't waste any of the experiences in our lives, ministry or otherwise, both good and bad! *Reclaiming the Joy of Ministry* offers a place for in-depth and engaging reflection, and provides a step by step pathway to design a personal intentional wellness plan. You'll find here the essence of the Grace Place Wellness Retreat!

Rev. Dr. Gregory S. Walton, President, Florida Georgia District LCMS

Anxiety, burnout, despair, and loneliness are too common in the lives of pastors and church workers. The illusion that church leaders are spiritual superheroes makes matters worse for them personally and in ministry. As he draws from his pastoral experience caring for hurting church servants and their spouses, the author shows concrete ways ministers of the Gospel can joyfully allow themselves to be cared for in order to properly care for others. This is not a how-to book about spiritual health, but an invitation to a lifelong journey of healing in Christ and through His Spirit. Every pastor and church worker who cares about their congregation, and every congregation that cares about their pastor and church workers, must read this book. A sober yet Gospel-filled approach to ministry for our hectic and anxious times.

Leopoldo A. Sánchez M., PhD
Director of the Center for Hispanic Studies, Concordia Seminary, St Louis

Reclaiming the Joy of Ministry is practical and grounded in scripture. Darrell Zimmerman and Grace Place Wellness Ministries have provided a process and model for church workers to plan and lead healthy, whole lives. Reclaiming the Joy of Ministry is a reminder that church workers are not alone. As they seek to put on their oxygen masks it is the very breath of our triune God giving them life and vitality so they may serve Him and His people.

Deaconess Tiffany Manor, Director, LCMS Life Ministry/Worker Wellness

Dr. Zimmerman's insight into church worker health and wellness is thoroughly precise and refreshing. His regular insertion of the prophet Elijah and his life experience reflect well the up and down cycles of ministry. He reminds us that when pastors or church workers serve from a posture of rest and are positively refreshed and renewed by God's means of grace and by those they love and trust, they resiliently withstand the roller coaster cycles of ministry. The Holy Spirit uses the crosses we bear to season and shape church workers to be more resilient and empathetic with those they serve. This book should be required reading for all future pastors, church workers and their spouses, enabling them to regularly check the pulse of their faith lives, bodily health, and relationships.

Rev. Timothy R. Puls (Ed.D.), Director of Alumni and Church Relations,
Concordia Theological Seminary, Fort Wayne

Softcover ISBN 978-1-7379478-0-6
e-book ISBN 978-1-7379478-1-3

10987654321

To my partners in ministry at
King of Kings, Salem, Peace,
Mount Calvary, and Salem (again).

"I always pray with joy
because of your partnership in the gospel,
from the first day until now."
Philippians 1:4-5

Acknowledgements

There is wisdom in the Body of Christ, imparted by the Spirit of the Living Word, Jesus. This book is testimony to the wisdom and compassion that thousands of church work couples at hundreds of Grace Place Wellness Retreats received and shared with one another in table conversations groups over the past two decades. Special thanks go to those who led our retreats for many years before my arrival, Rev. Darwin and Jan Karsten who led most of our retreats in the early years, and Rev. Dr. David and Kathy Ludwig, who passed me the baton in 2012, along with so much of their accumulated wisdom.

Heartfelt thanks also go to our ministry team during the time of writing, Beth McAnallen and Kathy Greffet for their patience during my frequent rants and encouragement as my faithful sounding boards.

The current volume, a revision of our first book *Reclaiming the Joy of Ministry*, would not be nearly as useful without the insights, critiques, and personal stories of the Commissioned Ministers who partnered with me: James Bradshaw, Education Executive of the Kansas District LCMS, DCE Rehema Kavugha, Deaconess Kristina Paul, DCEs Brian and Pam Amey, classroom educators Erica and John Spangler, retired Principal Dr. Joe Bordeaux, and most of all, Dr. Debra Afsten, Director of the DCE Program at Concordia University Chicago. Thanks, Debbie, for being brutally honest with an often clueless Pastor about the unique anxieties of "ministry from the second chair."

Contents

Foreword

Grace Place Wellness Ministries was born in the conversations of a physician and his patients in church work professions. While all people experience the effects of stress, there is a unique set of forces targeting the joy and fulfillment of both personal life and vocational service in church workers and, for that matter, their spouses. Simultaneously, literature arising from multiple church bodies reinforces the personal findings in the doctor's office: ministry is hard on professional church workers' and their families' health and wellness. And, when church worker wellbeing is adversely altered by a myriad of traumatic interactions, their effectiveness and longevity in their called profession is substantially limited. Often the end result is alarming: professional burnout.

What might stem the spiraling tide of loss from ministry? Grace Place Wellness Ministries chose a strategy steeped in the Scriptures and trumpeted by modern medicine: preventive care. Inspire and instill attitudes and behaviors which equip a ministry professional and spouse to be prepared for and proactive in addressing known challenges so common in ministry life. Provide a "pause point" for a church worker and spouse to step away from the daily friction part and parcel of vocation to be rested, renewed and reinvigorated for their journey. This "pause point" is not an "end point" but an opportunity, just like Elijah, to hear God's whisper and to be re-equipped for service, perhaps with a deeper understanding of the deleterious forces and armed with empowered tools for healthy living and service.

In the first twenty years of Grace Place Wellness Ministries, this took the form of week-long retreats for 12-20 couples held in beautiful and refreshing venues around the country. However, only a limited number of church workers and their families could access Grace Place Wellness Ministries' experiential education due to a host of circumstances. Frankly, the current pandemic accelerated a steadily growing realization: far more church workers and their spouses could benefit from this training and knowledge than the personal retreat method could effectively provide.

More recently, our current staff and board have been working on a delivery system for wholeness preventive care which we feel best provides wellness learnings to a larger and more diverse group of church work professionals. It begins with Rev. Dr. Zimmerman's comprehensive book which can lead a minister and their spouse into multiple avenues and resources (blogs, webinars, conferences) for self-directed realization, preparation and implementation of healthy ministry as well as on-going accountability.

We are assured that the Lord is caring directly for you, just as the Lord cared for his first church worker, Elijah. We encourage you to receive all the blessings of God's whisper as you seek to find rest, reassurance, restoration and resilience for a life of service to God's people. We pray for you joy in the journey.

John D. Eckrich, M.D.
Founder, Grace Place Wellness Ministries

Introduction

"I don't want to die in the pulpit," I said.

Since 2008 I've been part of a group of church workers and therapists who meet monthly to ask each other, "How are you doing?" It's neither just a polite greeting nor a rhetorical question. At my first session the group's facilitator asked me about "themes and concerns" in my life as part of my family of origin review. "I don't want to die in the pulpit" was the first thought that came to mind. I was serving my third congregation, a church with a long history of church worker burnout. One former pastor's family told me, "This church killed our dad in 1965. He was 54 years old." By the year 2000, about six years into my time there, I had begun to figure out why my predecessors had struggled so much, and I also began to realize that I was getting caught in the same trap. The demands of the ministry lifestyle and the anxieties of congregational life were taking a heavy toll on my spiritual life, on my family life, on my physical wellbeing, on my creativity, my energy and my passion for ministry.

Since my ordination in 1982, I had witnessed the spectacular views of ministry from 30,000 feet. Professional church workers in congregation and school ministry find tremendous joy in observing Jesus up close as he changes lives; healing broken hearts, filling people with hope, releasing them from the bonds of sin and death. Joy fuels ministry today the same way it fueled the ministries of apostles, martyrs and millions who served before us. I'd known the joy, but I'd also known the painful and sometimes sudden descent from the joy of Christian ministry into the downward spiral of despair that's far too common among professional church workers. All of my thirty years in parish life were spent in congregations with Christian schools. I lived the life of ministry alongside church work professionals of every stripe: Lutheran educators, musicians, Directors of Christian Education, Deaconesses, and Parish Nurses. I observed close hand that my experience was shared by every manner of church worker.

About mid-way through my parish experience, I found myself in a rapid descent from 30,000 feet and I was losing cabin pressure fast. The thought of leaving the ministry I loved, a thought that had surfaced occasionally in two previous parishes, was coming more and more frequently and it was getting harder to dismiss. At just the time I needed it most, an oxygen mask dropped from an overhead compartment. That breath of new life from the Spirit started me on a journey of recovery, a journey of re-creation and of renewed joy in ministry.

In the fall of 2000, my wife Carol and I were invited as last minute replacements on an experiment in clergy wellness, the first week long Grace Place Wellness retreat in the Colorado Rockies. Conceived in the heart of a medical doctor, Dr. John D. Eckrich of St. Louis, the retreat played off the flight attendant's instructions we had heard on our way to Aspen, "If you're traveling with someone who needs your assistance, put your own oxygen mask on first." Dr. Eckrich had treated hundreds of pastors, church workers, parochial school teachers, seminary students and their families over the years and was continually amazed at the levels of stress related illnesses they exhibited. After years of listening to the stories of church worker anxiety, and after prayer and dreaming big dreams for the Lord, he organized that first retreat. Led by Dr. Eckrich and our longtime friends and mentors, Rev. Dar and Jan Karsten, that pilot Grace Place Wellness retreat was the first time I had ever received permission to tend to my own spiritual, relational, emotional and physical needs in order to be more available to serve those same needs in others.[1] It had never occurred to me that caring for myself first would enhance my care for others.

Introduction

It was life changing for me and for Carol, and also for the church. Over the next ten years, as I learned the Lord's gospel-centered practices of preventive self-care, both I and the congregation became healthier, more joyful, more passionate about mission and outreach. Where I was once in danger of succumbing to the same forces that had destroyed the ministry careers of my predecessors, the Lord instilled in me a passion for hurting professional church workers and troubled congregations. The culmination of that journey to wellness came when I took training to serve as an Intentional Interim Pastor and asked my District President to send me to serve the most troubled churches in our region. I felt a new calling to share the lessons the church and I had learned along the way, lessons that every church and school ministry professional (and the churches they serve!) need to learn.

One day during my service as an Intentional Interim, twelve years and nearly 300 retreats after that first retreat in Aspen, Dr. Eckrich invited me to lunch and asked if I might be interested in serving alongside him as the first fulltime Program Director for Grace Place Wellness Ministries. These last nine years have provided the opportunity to share the lessons Carol and I learned, and to walk alongside thousands of professional church workers and their spouses as they learn to put their own oxygen masks in place.

Together we're discovering that ministry is a great and glorious calling, but very hard. We're learning that because ministry in church and school is the way of the cross and overwhelmed is a way of life for those who serve, no one should ever embark on this adventure alone. We're learning that joy is fuel for ministry, but the lifestyle and calling of ministry can threaten the joy of our own personal walks of faith with God, and it can threaten the joy of life in fellowship with those whom we love and serve. We're also learning that life in ministry can threaten the joy of Christian service! These lessons about the dangers of ministry, when taken to heart, have led us to conclude that since we suffer so many spiritual, emotional, relational and vocational wounds along the way, daily healing in the grace of Christ is essential. Every professional church worker who desires a long, productive, joyful career in ministry needs an intentional preventive wellness plan.

This book is an attempt to pass along some of those lessons with the hope that you might benefit from what I and thousands of others have learned through our trials and hardships. In fact, the lessons summarized in the previous paragraph serve as the outline for this book, the titles of the ten chapters that follow. I expect many of them are familiar territory for you already. Others might be brand new. All of them need to be taken to heart.

Our mission statement reads, *"Grace Place Wellness nurtures vitality and joy in ministry by inspiring and equipping church workers to lead healthy lives."* By "inspiring" we mean getting pastors, Christian educators and all church work professionals to realize that helping others with their oxygen masks without first tending to their own is foolishness of the worst kind. Tragically, it seems to be an occupational hazard for every category of church work professional. In the chapters that follow, we'll take a look at why that happens so often. By "equipping" we mean learning the skills required to do regular self-assessments and finding answers to the question, "How am I doing, spiritually, relationally and vocationally?"

If at the end of the Ten Lessons that follow you are led to develop and pursue a preventive self-care plan to address your own particular situation, I'll introduce you to our equipping resource, the *Reclaiming the Joy of Ministry* Workbook Series, available through our website at **GracePlaceWellness.org**. We're still learning. The current version of the workbook is filled with the latest research and resources to guide you as you seek the Lord's healing touch; the renewal and refreshment for service in the church and the Christian school that only God can provide.

Introduction

DARRELL'S POINT OF VIEW

Early on in this text you'll recognize my background as an ordained minister of The Lutheran Church Missouri Synod. Martin Luther made more than his share of blunders in his walk of faith and service. I'm convinced that his understanding of the enormity of the power of the gospel to heal and to save comes from his inability to overcome his failures by his own wisdom and strength. He knew the greatness of God so well because he knew his own weakness. That puts me in good company. I find in Luther's thought and in the Confessional writings of the Lutheran Church great wisdom for any disciple of Jesus seeking a fuller and richer life of faith and service. (It's also the doctrinal material I know the best, so naturally I quote it the most!) If you are from a different Christian tradition, I trust you to apply these lessons from your own theological perspective, but I believe you'll find Luther's insight helpful.

The professional church workers of The LCMS are categorized as either "Ordained" or "Commissioned" ministers: ordained pastors and the other commissioned ministerial offices adjunct to the pastoral office such as Deaconesses, Parochial School Teachers, Directors of Christian Education, Music and Outreach, etc. Your faith tradition may define these roles differently. Throughout the book, I'll most often use the term "church workers" to refer to the broad spectrum of professionals in both parish ministry and the ministry of Christian schools. The work that we do together in church and school I will refer to as "ministry." Whether ordained or commissioned, we are all in ministry. This book is a revision of my first book, *Reclaiming the Joy of Ministry* that was primarily directed toward ordained pastors. This volume is laced through with insights from those who have walked in your shoes and have endured the challenges of ministry that are unique to non-ordained church work professionals. I'll include my observations from my thirty years of working closely with both ordained and commissioned ministers in team ministry settings in churches and Lutheran schools. Each congregation that I served was affiliated with Christian elementary and high schools and I know from experience that few church workers are expected to accomplish so much with such limited resources as Christian educators.

Church workers who are not married frequently endure insensitivity to their lifestyle that most church leaders, (and many of their fellow servants in ministry), do not fully appreciate. The specific anxieties of ministry unique to single church workers can be a particularly strong force in diminishing the joy of a life in ministry. We'll be talking about the burdens of the ministry lifestyle throughout; single church workers are often saddled with burdens that are unjust and inappropriate. It's my hope that unmarried church workers studying Reclaiming the Joy will seek out peers in ministry who do understand with whom they can process the Lessons found here in a way most beneficial to their calling.

Married church workers know that our spouses play a critical role in the wellbeing of their beloved. Church worker's husbands and wives are often more attuned to the stresses that their loved ones are enduring than we are. I'm convinced that this book would have a far greater impact if church worker's spouses would read it first. They'd respond the way Carol did at that first retreat, poking me under the table during the conversations about church worker burnout and whispering at me, "That's YOU!" If you are married to a parochial school teacher or church work professional, I consider you a partner in our effort at Grace Place Wellness Ministries to get those oxygen masks firmly planted on the faces of those on whom we all depend! God bless you as you offer encouragement, guidance and a sense of urgency to the one you love to find the grace they need.

The objectives of all Grace Place Wellness programming drive this volume as well. We have three heartfelt desires for every church worker. First, we want you to have the wisdom and awareness to recognize the multi-faceted ways that a life in ministry negatively affects your own spiritual, emotional, relational, physical, intellectual, financial and vocational lives. We want you to have the skills necessary to assess how that brokenness has impacted your effectiveness as a disciple of Christ and as a called servant in the Church. We want you to understand why you're hurting.

Second, it's our hope that every professional church worker would know where to turn to find healing and grace for restoration by the power of the gospel and to have the humility of spirit to pause from striving forward in ministry under their own power and instead avail themselves of strength from on high. Our hope is that every church worker in distress will find daily healing by the grace and mercy of God and be put back on the journey to the spiritual, relational and vocational wholeness that God intends.

Third, since the vast majority of professional church workers work in team ministry settings, which present both unique joys and unique challenges, we hope that careful study of this volume together in your team will help enhance the unity and cooperation that is so essential for team ministry. As the Apostles themselves discovered, our partners in the work of the kingdom can be both a burden and a blessing, but the Lord is always present among his people, gathering us from disparate backgrounds and binding us together as one in the unity of his body to serve as his hands and feet, eyes and ears. A team ministry discussion guide is included at the end of each of the Ten Lessons.

And finally, it's our dream for the body of Christ that church work professionals who have themselves received the grace of Christ in their own lives will be better able to lead their congregations and schools to be places of healing. When called workers and the family of God together find strength to continue on despite our common brokenness, we more effectively share the good news of a Savior's love to the broken and hurting people of our communities.

Reclaiming the Joy of a Church Vocation

This world is broken, as are all of us who journey here. Recent world events have dramatically reshaped the very nature of our calling. We're discovering day by day how different it is to do what church workers do. And it's more challenging than ever for ministry teams to flourish in their kingdom service together. My prayer is that this book will help inspire and equip you to make healthy choices for your own wellbeing as a teacher, a leader, a servant of the gospel, choices that will also influence those around you and enhance your service together. I pray that you will be better equipped to serve your community with vitality and joy.

Deaconess Kris Paul summarized for us very well why this book was necessary. She told me, "There's something unique to the ministry experience of 'non-pastors': we are not as central to the public ministry in the life of the church as pastors are, but we're not exactly a part of the regular fellowship of the congregation either. We don't take all the hits the Pastor takes, but we do not always receive the love the Pastor does either. It is sometimes a sort of 'stagehand' ministry — which makes it even more important that we find time to be with ministry crew for joy and support."

Well said, Kris. It's our hope that as you and those with whom you serve in ministry study and discuss *Reclaiming the Joy of a Church Vocation* you will find that joy and support.

I'm convinced that even in your trials, God is at work in you for good, even though the Lord's work is seldom completed suddenly, in a flash. Our God is a God of changing seasons, working slowly, deliberately, unfolding his purposes and working his works of transformation and new life at his own pace. In Matthew 13 Jesus taught the Parable of the Leaven, the yeast that slowly, eventually works its way through the whole lump of dough. Luther taught that the work our gracious God is doing in your life and in mine is much like that leaven.

Introduction

The new leaven is the faith and grace of the Spirit. It does not leaven the whole lump at once, but gently, and gradually, we become like this new leaven and eventually, a bread of God. This life, therefore, is not godliness but the process of becoming godly, not health but getting well, not being but becoming, not rest but exercise. We are not now what we shall be, but we are on the way. The process is not yet finished, but it is actively going on. This is not the goal but it is the right road. At present, everything does not gleam and sparkle, but everything is being cleansed.[2]

I hope and pray that the Lessons contained here will be a blessing to you on your journey!

Pentecost, 2021

Reclaiming the Joy of Team Ministry

HOW LEAD PASTORS AND SCHOOL ADMINISTRATORS CAN USE THIS BOOK TO BUILD A FLOURISHING TEAM.

We at Grace Place Wellness Ministries are convinced that in ministry settings where church and school staff flourish, certain key essentials are in place:

▸ Team leaders (e.g. Lead Pastors and School Administrators) take the lead in creating the supportive, caring environment church workers need to survive and thrive in ministry.

▸ The unity that Christ gives to his body, the Church, is lived out in practical ways that display a mutual trust, respect, and love for one another.

▸ Communication is open and honest.

▸ Conflict is dealt with by sincere confession and freely offered forgiveness.

▸ Every member of the team assumes their responsibility for the team's wellness.

▸ The team has and follows an intentional plan for everyone's wellness.

Reclaiming the Joy of a Church Vocation is designed specifically to help ministry team leaders guide their partners in ministry into the full, rich, (sometimes awkward and painful), conversations that will lead to healing and to changes in team behavior, changes that help create the supportive environment where everyone flourishes in ministry.

As you read, study, reflect on, and discuss together each of the Ten Lessons, we suggest the following:

▶ Set a schedule and get everyone's commitment to study the Ten Lessons together, either in regular staff/faculty meetings or in a retreat setting.

▶ Engage the whole team in prayer for your time of growth. This is God's kingdom work.

▶ Expect every member of the team to complete the "Not Finished Yet" guide at the end of each Lesson on their own in preparation for your group conversations.

▶ Use the "Ministry Team Conversation Starters" to do just that: start the conversation. Be open to the Spirit leading you into the conversation that your team needs to have. Every team in its own unique setting will have different issues to discuss. Find them.

▶ Remember that your wellness is a matter of spiritual warfare. Satan wants your team to stay stuck in unhealthy places. On the other side of tough conversations, Jesus brings healing and joy.

▶ Every team has issues that are so emotionally charged that they avoid discussing them as they should. Show enough faith in the Lord of the Church, and in one another, to tackle the tough topics together.

▶ Seek outside guidance to help address your wellness concerns when necessary.

▶ Be intentional about developing a plan to find healing for the past and to develop new strategies for the future as you move forward in healthier ways. You'll find guidance to get started in Lessons Nine and Ten.

- ▸ Grace Place Wellness Ministries has developed other resources to guide you in your wellness journey.

- ▸ *Reclaiming the Joy of Ministry: The Grace Place Way to Church Worker Wellness* is a more compete study of the topic, specifically directed toward ordained clergy. Pastors leading their teams in a study of the present volume would be enriched by addressing their own wellness through a study of our previous book.

- ▸ The *Reclaiming the Joy of Ministry* Workbook Series is a guide for developing a personal wellness plan. Eight separate volumes are designed to lead your personal reflection on the biblical themes of wellness as they relate to Baptismal, Spiritual, Relational, Intellectual, Emotional, Vocational, Physical, and Financial Wellness. You may also find them helpful as an additional resource and useful guide to develop a team wellness plan.

You can find more information about these and other Grace Place Wellness resources and programs at our website, **GracePlaceWellness.org**.

Prolog: A Church Worker's Plea

O God,

I was so humbled when you called. A sinner like me? With my unclean lips? I was sure you had the wrong person, but I heard your call and I followed because the need is so great and I just want everyone to know your love the way I do.

I've known so much joy sharing Jesus, but I had no idea that it could be so hard.

I've started to wonder again if you really did call the right person. I've got so many questions, questions I never considered before we started this adventure together.

How can I serve with all my heart and still have time for a life of my own and a life with my family?

How can I ever live up to the expectations the church places on me?

How can I keep up this pace for even another year or two? It seems the harder I try, the worse it gets.

I wish I had someone that I could talk to, to tell how I could really use some help. I've seen how people in ministry talk about each other. Is it safe to tell anyone I work with how much I'm struggling? I bless others, but I need a blessing. I listen all day long, but who would listen to me?

I teach others about the way of love, joy and peace, but wonder if I'm starting to lose my own way.

I need your help, Lord. I need your healing touch. My relationships are broken. My emotions are broken. My finances and my body are broken.

I've seen others in ministry crash and burn and I'm afraid of what might happen to me. We've been to the mountaintop together, haven't we, Lord? And we've been through the valleys. I want to continue on the next part of the journey, and the next, and the next, but I'll need to find a place to be replenished, restored, and renewed along the way.

A place called Grace.

I

LESSON ONE

Ministry Is Great, but Hard

IT WAS A GOOD DAY TO BE A PROPHET. A great day to be a prophet. It might possibly be the best day ever for a called worker in God's kingdom. Ever.

I'm sure you remember the scene well. It was a defining moment for the nation of Israel and for the Lord's servant, Elijah. After a couple of bulls were prepped for incineration on the top of Mount Carmel, the prophets of Baal, outnumbering Elijah 850 to one, took the first whack. Elijah must have been beaming as he spent the greater portion of the day sarcastically ridiculing the false prophets and mocking their impotent god. Their dancing, their shouting and even their bloody pleas of "We're dying down here!" couldn't rouse Baal's attention. "Maybe he's sleeping, or on vacation, or 'indisposed.' Oh, you poor little bleeding prophets! Too bad your god can't help you" (see 1 Kings 18:27).

And then it was Elijah's turn, because it was God's turn. After drenching the tinderbox so there would be no post-firestorm inquiry, Elijah humbly prayed, "Dear Lord, you show them who is God." And in an instant, the Lord did. It was a great day to be a worker in God's kingdom. Fire fell from the sky.

Altar, wood, ox, and water were consumed in a flash. Prophets were chased down and executed. It was an unmatched day of victory for the Lord, for his Word of truth and for his humble servant, Elijah. It was a day for joy and you'd have every reason to expect that the next day would be a day for rest, for celebration, and for basking once again in the joy of God's goodness.

Or so you would think.

The rapturous celebration of victory in the aftermath of 1 Kings 18 should be first on the "Top Ten Reasons to Become a Professional Church Worker" list, but it never happened. What did happen next serves instead as the perfect illustration for the first lesson that church workers need to learn on their journey to long, productive and joy-filled years of service in God's kingdom: "Ministry is great, but hard." It's a painful paradox, but it's true, and the sooner we take this lesson to heart, the more likely we'll be to survive and even thrive in the face of the challenges of church work. Sadly, although Elijah had known for some time how **great** the joys of ministry could be, he seemed unaware of just how **hard** the call can be.

> Although Elijah had known for some time how great the joys of ministry could be, he seemed unaware of just how hard the call can be.

They don't teach you this in Sunday School, but by the fourth verse of the next chapter, Elijah had given up all hope, resigned from ministry and begged God to take his life. Chapter 19 of 1 Kings is one of the earliest and one of the best depictions in the Bible of the hazards of a life in ministry.

Elijah is the "poster boy" for the way that church workers, if they're not attentive to their wellbeing, can run into serious trouble. Elijah was about to make ministry much harder on himself than God intends it to be. The surprising revelation that ministry would be both great and hard would lead him on a journey down the mountain and into the wilderness, a journey into anxiety, exhaustion, loneliness and despair, and then finally, by the grace of God, to a path back out of the valley and into service in God's kingdom again.

Let's resume the story back on the top of Mount Carmel. After the fire of God fell from the sky, Elijah looked around and certainly had plenty of reason to think that he was witnessing a clean sweep, a total victory for Yahweh, God of Israel. This, of course, is what he had prayed for just moments earlier. "O Lord, God of Abraham, Isaac and Israel, let it be known today that you are God in Israel..." (1 Kings 18:36). Great prayer! All the glory goes to God, right? But there's a hint in the next petition that something may have started to go awry. Elijah continued, "...and [let it be known today] that I am your servant and have done all these things at your command."

Careful, Elijah. That sounds like a desire for personal vindication. To this point, he seems to have kept his ego, his foolish pride, out of the equation. Ministry is great when it's all about the advancement of the kingdom of God, the Lord's reign in the hearts and lives of people. But service in church and school gets hard when it starts to become all about the church worker.

It's easy to see how Elijah could have gotten caught up in the groundswell of what he saw on the mountaintop. After fire fell from heaven, the people shouted, "The Lord, he is God! The Lord, he is God!" The populace was converted, but what about the potentate? If wicked King Ahab were to repent and lead the nation to follow, Elijah would be vindicated and honored as the spiritual leader of the nation's revival. It's clear from the text that Elijah thought Ahab was thoroughly impressed and that a national reformation was beginning to take shape.[3] Ahab had not resisted the extermination of the failed prophets. By the next morning Elijah had become the king's valet, encouraging him to eat and drink before the victory procession back to the palace. He became the king's personal meteorologist, warning him to beat the rush hour downpour and get his chariot moving. Elijah became Ahab's vanguard, drum major and escort, running for twenty-seven miles before the king on his way back to the palace in Jezreel. Elijah seems to be thinking, "Now they're going to know who the prophet of the Lord is! This ministry stuff is great, and I'm the miracle worker leading the biggest revival in the history of God's chosen people!"

Meanwhile back at the palace, faithless Queen Jezebel was most likely watching her favorite storm god, Baal, unleash his victory flood (so she thinks) after putting that "troubler of Israel" Elijah in his place. The king's procession arrived home to meet the unlovely and ungracious Queen Jezebel, and that's when it all started to unravel. It was the day after the greatest day ever, and it started to turn into the worst day a church worker ever had. Ahab told Jezebel everything that had transpired, and she didn't like it. She ordered the prophet's execution. "Today!"

When Elijah heard he was under the death sentence, he took off running south and didn't stop until leaving Israel, running the whole length of Judah and collapsing completely broken, curled up under a broom tree in the wilderness of Beersheba, desperately in need of rest and the healing touch of God's grace.

What just happened?

When the Sunday School version of Elijah makes him out to be one of the Great Heroes of the Bible, we miss the point of the story; of the entire Bible, actually. There's only one Hero in God's salvation history. Sometimes we forget that.

When Elijah forgot, he paid a tremendous spiritual, emotional, vocational and physical price for his failure.

The long journey to Beersheba gave him plenty of time to wonder to himself just what had happened. If he's like most of us ("Elijah was a man just like us," James 5:17), he used the time to play The Blame Game. "It's the devil's fault!" (No, he was just proven impotent on the mountain). "It's the people's fault!" (No, there's a revival underway). "I wasn't prepared for this in school!" (No, church worker training never prepared anyone for everything). "It's God's fault! Where was he when I needed him?" (We'll get to that in a minute). Elijah looked everywhere to find someone to blame except the one place he should have looked first: in the mirror.

Well, back at the broom tree, the angel of the Lord came to Elijah, woke him up with a gentle touch, refreshed him with warm baked bread and a long drink of cool water and then, (after another nap), woke him up once again and sent him on retreat. After being refreshed with a miraculously sustaining meal, Elijah traveled forty days and forty nights deeper into the wilderness to meet with God on the mountain of the Lord, Mount Horeb, also known as Mount Sinai, the place where God met with Moses.

It was lesson time for Elijah. Where was God in this? He was about to find out.

There they were again, Elijah and Yahweh on another mountaintop. Mount Carmel had been a very public battleground for the heart of a nation. What Elijah had failed to see was that there was another more personal battle raging at the same time. The second battle was the spiritual warfare in the heart of the Lord's servant, and Elijah was losing the battle. So the Lord engaged Elijah in a spiritual renewal retreat that would lead to his healing and to his restoration back into a life of joyful ministry.

I have a tendency to overthink my situation when things start to go wrong. My mind starts churning through every permutation of Murphy's Law. Apparently Elijah shared the same tendency. After another time of rest in a cave on the mountain of the Lord, a word came to him asking, "What are you doing here, Elijah?" (1 Kings 19:9). As a natural over-thinker, he had a soliloquy all prepared, a litany of his tale of woe as a faithful servant of the Word whose joy in ministry had run out. Elijah said, "I have been very zealous for the Lord God Almighty. The Israelites have rejected your covenant, broken down your altars, and put your prophets to death with the sword. I am the only one left, and now they are trying to kill me too" (1 Kings 19:10). Uh-oh, Elijah. Remember his prayer for personal vindication? He's done it again. Notice why Elijah thought he was on retreat: his little speech began and ended with "me." "I'm doing a great job! They don't come more zealous than this guy. I don't see anyone else toughing it out for three years eating bread and water. I've put up with more insults and disrespect and with more unresponsive church members than anyone in Israel, and if that's not enough, now they want to kill me for it. I deserve better than this!"

It's heartbreaking to hear how disillusioned about ministry Elijah had become, but (and one of the greatest words in the Bible is "but," isn't it?) the Lord is a God of healing and hope and he had a great blessing in store for his servant. Elijah had come to the retreat out of resentment and hurt, wanting answers and wanting vindication. Yahweh wanted him there to learn and grow.

Elijah had fallen prey to Satan's attack and was losing the spiritual battle that could potentially drive him out of ministry. There in the cave on the mountain, Elijah fell for one of the devil's nastiest, but most effective arguments: "You can't do this, Elijah." His earlier unquestioned confidence in Yahweh's ability to feed the starving, raise the dead and shut off the nation's rainfall for three years was supplanted by his growing awareness that he was in way over his head. Maybe he fully realized how helpless he was against the forces of evil and decided that he had no future in ministry. If so, he was right. He was in way over his head.

> **Maybe he believed the other lie, "Elijah, you can do this!"**

It could be, however, that Elijah had previously fallen victim to one of Satan's even more insidious strategies in his spiritual warfare against church workers. Maybe he believed the other lie, "Elijah, you can do this!" It's the same trick that the devil would try to use on Jesus in a different wilderness centuries later. Elijah's trouble began when his human pride and self-centeredness crept in and began to misplace his confidence and trust in the Lord alone. It's so ironic because Elijah's name literally means, "The Lord is my God!"

There was only one correct answer in The Blame Game. Elijah's problem was... Elijah!

But because he is faithful, God had a plan to bring Elijah through the wilderness of despair, loneliness and fear, back to a place of humility, faith and victory. Part of the plan was to give the prophet a Moses-sized theophany of the Lord's way of working in the hearts of his chosen servants.

God called Elijah to stand at the mouth of the cave to witness his presence passing by, much as Moses had on the same mountain. There was a lesson to be learned, and it wouldn't come easy. Elijah was about to discover the mysterious ways of the Lord, ways that were far different than Elijah was expecting. As he stood there on the Mountain of the Lord, Elijah didn't find God in the usual places: he wasn't found in the hurricane force wind that shattered Sinai's boulders, or in the earthquake or the wildfire that followed. Elijah met God in the life-renewing Word whispered in his ear. The second time it was a soft voice asking the same question as before, "What are you doing here, Elijah?" (1 Kings 19:13). Now this is interesting. In a classic over-thinker's response to the Lord's compassionate inquiry, the prophet recited in verse fourteen exactly verbatim, word for word, the litany of misery he had just stated in verse ten: "I have been very zealous for the Lord God Almighty. The Israelites have rejected your covenant, broken down your altars, and put your prophets to death with the sword. I am the only one left, and now they are trying to kill me too." Just like the first time, it was still mostly about Elijah.

It was a good lament, an outpouring of misery that was an important part of Elijah's healing. The Lord's therapeutic renewal began with Elijah's heart-felt, though inaccurate, expression of grief and despair. The healing power of the gospel comes only after the full burden of sin has been exposed. In a sense, the prophet was right about one thing: it was time for him to die, but not the way he had expressed it earlier. The journey to a new wisdom and a new vitality and joy in ministry comes when our old sinful nature is drowned and dies, when all of our internalized lies, our corrupted understanding of ourselves, are finally put to death so that God can work in us a miracle of renewal and raise us up to a new life. In both the Old Testament and the New Testament, God works the same way. I really like how Paul explains it to the Ephesians. "You were taught, with regard to your former way of life, to put off your old self, which is being corrupted by its deceitful desires; to be made new in the attitude of your minds; and to put on the new self, created to be like God in true righteousness and holiness" (Ephesians 4:22-24). It was time for the old Elijah to die, to be made new, and to rise again.

That's when the Lord delivered the biggest surprise of all. He wasn't through with Elijah just yet. In the midst of his brokenness, the Lord God came and brought healing by the restoring power of the Word of hope. First, God shattered Elijah's well-rehearsed discourse of inaccurate negative self-talk with words of divine law, straightening out the crooked paths of the lies Elijah was telling himself. Elijah was wrong about the covenant. The covenant with Israel continued despite the corruption in the royal palace and God would be establishing new leadership soon, in his own time and in his own way, and certainly not according to Elijah's plan. And Elijah was wrong about the prophets, too. The prophets, while decimated, were still alive and functioning (see 1 Kings 18:13).

And finally there came a word of promise and gospel. "You're not alone, Elijah. I have a partner for you, Elisha, not to mention the seven thousand in Israel you've forgotten about who haven't bowed down to the false gods. And your work is not yet done because my work is not yet done. I'll have victory over evil kings and their empires and over Satan and his false prophets. Now go back the way you came. You're back in business. I have plans for you because my kingdom work is not yet complete" (see 1 Kings 19:15-18).

Lesson One on the journey to a long and vibrant career in church work says, "Ministry is great, but hard." What Elijah (and all who follow him) had to learn was that ministry is great because God is great. The only Hero in the Bible is the One who established his covenant of grace with Abraham and with Moses and with David to rescue the world from sin and death by sending the Messiah, his Son. That salvation history was going to unfold according to the Lord's plan, not according to Elijah's. Revival, reformation, the fall of evil kings and queens would happen according to God's timing and plan and no one else's. And Elijah also needed to learn that ministry is hard because we make it hard. When our expectations of vindication and glory run counter to God's intent, we always suffer disappointment, discouragement and hardship. It happens over and over again because it's our nature to seek the glory and avoid the burden of the cross-bearing to which we are called.

The journey to wisdom and church worker wellness nearly always takes us down the treacherous path of sinful pride and foolish mistakes. It's our nature and it's the history of all who've gone before us. Before we learn the way of humble obedience, we make lots of mistakes. Just ask Abraham, Moses, David, Peter, (shall I go on?) As you continue reading, you'll hear about a few of my blunders. The good news for church work professionals is that God is faithful and repeatedly calls us to put off the old, to be made new by forgiveness and mercy, and to put on the new, making more and more of the wise choices that help us face, refreshed and renewed, the challenges and burdens of the life of ministry that we love so dearly.

So why do we love it so much? Why do we and thousands of our peers in school and church ministry continue on, riding both the highs and the lows of this calling, believing that this journey fraught with peril is worth the cost? I believe it's because as hard as a life in ministry can be, the joy of watching

> As hard as a life in ministry can be, the joy watching Jesus Christ show up and transform lives is even greater!

Jesus Christ show up and transform lives is even greater! That's Lesson One: Ministry is great, but hard.

I'm reminded of a favorite scene from a movie that always makes me think of Jesus offering words of encouragement to his disciples. It's a speech made by Jimmy Dugan, Manager of the Rockford Peaches of the All-American Girls' Professional Baseball League, Tom Hanks' character in the movie "A League of Their Own." He's talking about how great the game of baseball is, but there's wisdom for church workers in what he said. When star player Dottie Hinson, played by Geena Davis, announced that she was quitting the team because, "It just got too hard," Dugan at first turned away in disgust, then he marched right back to Dottie and through gritted teeth in his deepest, most serious tone, told her, "It's supposed to be hard. If it wasn't hard, everyone would do it. The hard is what makes it great."

The same could be said about following Jesus into a life in ministry. It is hard; but the hard is what makes it great. In spite of ourselves and the myriad ways we make it so hard, Jesus keeps showing up and making it great. That's Lesson One in the journey toward wellness, and the sooner a professional church worker takes this lesson to heart, the sooner that worker moves toward the wholeness, peace and joy that God has planned for his kingdom workers.

.

NOT FINISHED YET!

Take a few minutes to consider whether Lesson One, "Ministry is great, but hard" is a lesson about ministry that you've taken to heart.

» What did you read in this chapter that resonates most deeply? What made you say to yourself, "That's really true!"?

quote by Tom Hanks in A League of Their Own.

» How would you phrase Lesson One differently?

Our ministry is worth the negative pulls.

» What did Darrell not discuss in this chapter that really could have been mentioned?

more of how we as Church workers could relate to Elijah more.

» If this is a lesson you've already learned from your own experience, when did you first discover that it was true?

During Covid 19 closure

» What needs your further contemplation before moving on to the next chapter?

Self reflection of what joys I miss in my teaching.

MINISTRY TEAM CONVERSATION STARTERS FOR LESSON ONE

» Share with the other members of your ministry team what you feel is great about your ministry. *Being able to make learning fun and seeing the growth of my students*

» When did you first realize how hard a life in ministry can be? *This year has really knocked me down.*

» Do you remember the first time you heard of a friend leaving their ministry? What were your thoughts? *Yes, Kirsten to be a stay at home mom and I was worried for her.*

» Share a time when you were ready to give up on the call to ministry. What prompted your thoughts? What helped you work through that time? *This year, with David + Coworkers, my parents and other students from past and future.*

» How many heroes are there in the Bible? What comfort does that give you? *1 hero - Jesus and brings me so much comfort knowing He's got my plans for me.*

» Discuss what Jimmy Dugan said to Dottie Henson: "It's supposed to be hard. If it wasn't hard, anyone could do it. It's the hard that makes it great." *Lutheran teaching isn't for everyone. It's going to be tough to stand out from others and build the strongest leaders for life.*

LESSON TWO

Because Ministry Is the Way of the Cross

WE'RE ALL A BIT LIKE ELIJAH. Actually, we're a lot like Elijah. Being used as an instrument of the Lord to share his Word of law and gospel can be tremendously exhilarating and richly rewarding.

It can also be discouraging and exhausting.

I've asked thousands of teachers and parish professionals, "How are you doing? How is life in ministry these days?" If I could, I'd ask you the same, even though I know there's no way to predict how you might answer. We're all like Elijah, somewhere along the winding road that has a countless number of both peaks and valleys.

In our work at Grace Place Wellness Ministries we hear expressions of discouragement from church workers all the time, people who sound a bit like they're sitting under the broom tree. Have you ever, maybe recently, had any of the feelings that your peers have expressed while on one of our retreats?

- ▶ "I bless others, but I could use a blessing myself."

- ▶ "People come to me for healing, but I'm as broken as anybody else."

- ▶ "I'm tired and I can't go on. I'm all used up."

- ▶ "I'm not who people think I am."

- ▶ "The reality of this work is not like the dream."

- ▶ "Going into church work was a mistake."

- ▶ "Teaching has become only a job."

- ▶ "Ministry is hurting my family life."

- ▶ "Ministry is hurting my faith life."

- ▶ "My life is a complaint box."

- ▶ "I am the chief piñata."

Because we serve Elijah's God, there is always hope for a new beginning. It's been our privilege at Grace Place Wellness to see the Lord grant that gift through our renewal retreats over and over and over again, hundreds and thousands of times. A Christian school administrator and his wife expressed it beautifully not long ago: "We came battle worn, completely exhausted and depleted. We're leaving today physically rested, and spiritually and emotionally nurtured." There is hope when faced with periods of doubt, and even despair, hope that God can restore and send us back to the harvest fields. We continue to hear over and over again expressions of joy in ministry like,

- ▶ "I consistently and regularly experience tremendous joy in my calling."

- ▶ "I can't imagine spending my life doing anything else."

▶ "Through every challenge, God has been faithful. He always provides."

▶ "What a privilege to be called into this wonderful work!"

I don't know where you are in your ministry right now. You might be riding high on Mount Carmel and can't even imagine a day when you won't feel enthusiasm for the work that lies ahead. On the other hand maybe you're discouraged, lying low in a cave on Mount Horeb, unable to imagine that the days of your passion for ministry will ever return. Maybe you can't quite tell if you're at a high point or a low point because you've been thrown so high and brought so low on the roller coaster ride of the peaks and valleys of ministry lately that you can't tell how you feel. But it begs a question that professional church workers often find themselves asking: "Why? Why does ministry have to be so hard?"

Nearly every experienced church worker has taken the Elijah journey and has learned that a life in Christian ministry can be a paradox of emotions: times of joy and times of anxiety all jumbled together. It's a story of the struggle that is inherent to a life in kingdom service. It's Lesson Two on the journey to wellness: ministry is great, but hard, "Because it's the way of the cross."

> **Nearly every experienced church worker has taken the Elijah journey.**

WHY DIDN'T SOMEONE TELL ME?

The generation of church workers before us could have warned us, but maybe they (like us) were afraid to admit how hard it can be. Most of us are pretty good at hiding the toll that this calling can take, and maybe our own models for church work as we were growing up were pretty good at doing the same thing. Maybe the urgency to recruit young people into church work careers contributed to that temptation to present ministry as all glory and joy without the counterbalancing truth of the crosses. It's probably a good thing that many of us had no idea how demanding the call can be or we might not have signed up in the first place!

It doesn't take long for most professional church workers in their first assignment to discover that the tasks of church and school ministry are never ending. No matter how many long hours of effort are given in a day or in a week, there are always more families to be visited, more programs to be developed, more meetings to be attended. The unending stream of one week after the next on much the same schedule is physically exhausting.

As demanding as the job can be physically, a ministry calling can be even more taxing emotionally, and that catches many of us off guard. Listening compassionately to the cares and concerns of others is more emotionally exhausting than we're prepared for. Church workers who scurry after everyone else's needs without tending to their own wellbeing often find themselves under broom trees.

There's a relational price that is often required of people in church work professions also. Elijah's lament under the broom tree indicates the depths of loneliness and isolation he was experiencing. Tending to the needs of our own families as well as the needs of those we serve can be a delicate balancing act and a breeding ground for misunderstanding and hurt feelings at home and resentment at church. People in ministry are caught in a triangle of the pull toward tending to their own needs, or serving their own family as a spouse and as a parent, and the equally strong tug to serve the church's families. The needs of the one are often resented by the other. Financial stress only adds to the tension between church and home.

Maybe most surprising to church workers is the toll that is sometimes taken on their own personal spiritual life. It's a tragic paradox that those called to enrich the spiritual lives of others should suffer depletion in their own walk with the Lord. Elijah walked closely with God, but still found himself desperately in need of the renewing Word of the Lord. His collapse should serve as a warning to everyone in ministry that even the richest and most rewarding experiences of ministry can lead to times of despair and hopelessness if we're not prepared.

JESUS TOLD US

I expect you might be reading this book because you've known what Elijah knew: this life in Christian service can grind a person down. Jesus taught the disciples that the way of Christian leadership would be far more cross than glory. I almost hate to say what comes next, because on the surface it sounds so insensitive, but it needs to be said. In what appears at first to be the most uncaring and inconsiderate words that Jesus ever spoke, we find the key to enduring through the challenging times that God's children have always experienced. Right after the eight "blesseds" of the Beatitudes, those words of encouragement Jesus spoke to begin his Sermon on the Mount, our Lord continued, shifting his pronoun from "blessed are they" to "blessed are you." "Blessed are you when people insult you, persecute you and falsely say all kinds of evil against you because of me. Rejoice and be glad, because great is your reward in heaven, for in the same way they persecuted the prophets who were before you" (Matthew 5:11-12). We stand in the long line of the faithful who have borne the cares of ministry before us; the prophets, the apostles, the martyrs of the faith. We hold to the same hope of reward in heaven, and in the midst of this time of the cross, with the hope of glory to come, God gives the gift that carries us through, little glimpses of the perfect joy that lies before us that provides us with strength to continue on.

Cross bearing is a lesson clearly taught throughout the scriptures. Joseph learned it. Abraham and Sarah learned it. The judges, the good kings and the prophets all learned it. Esther and Ezra and Nehemiah learned it too. Life with God is the way of the cross, but that's not something we want to hear and it's not an easy lesson to get through our thick skulls.

An ancient African proverb states, "Smooth seas do not make skillful sailors." According to Luther, God is recognized for his work in our lives not in those times and places where everything is smooth sailing and we feel like we're doing just fine. God is recognized more clearly in the times of struggle as we face the burdens and cares of our fallen humanity. It's in the times of darkness that we turn to the light of Christ. In those darkest times, we're tempted to doubt God's faithfulness and cry out, "Where is God in this?" Where he is constitutes the wonder and surprising beauty of the gospel. He's in the last place we'd expect. The hidden God is most clearly displayed in the suffering and death of Jesus on the cross. It's at the foot of the cross of Christ that we finally discover our absolute inability to save ourselves and God's infinite power and love to save the unredeemable. And this is the mystery: it's on display in his own suffering and death.

MINISTRY PARADOX: THE STRUGGLE AND THE JOY

It's a curious thing about life in ministry: just when you think that it has to be the greatest of all possible callings on earth, you're reminded that it can be incredibly, and often even unbearably, hard. C. F. W. Walther understood the nature of the paradox of joy in the midst of struggle. During his time as a pastor, seminary professor and denominational president, he endured episodes of personal anxiety and depression. As a leader in the church he dealt with conflict, betrayal, slander, doctrinal controversy, gossip and threats of rebellion; you know, the usual ministry stuff. Through it all, Walther continually affirmed that even though a life of service in the Church is a life of struggle and hardship, ministers of the gospel are holders of the most glorious office this world has ever known. In his lectures to seminary students about life in ministry, Walther once said,

> Yea, I am forced to say that, if the holy angels, who have been confirmed in eternal bliss, were capable of envy, they would, even in their state of celestial glory, unquestionably envy every teacher of the Gospel. For all that is recorded concerning [the angels] in Holy Scripture does not equal the greatness of the office of teachers and preachers, in which [we] become helpers in the task of bringing fallen creatures back to their Creator."[4]

That's quite an image, isn't it? I don't know if what he suggests about the angels and their jealousy is true or not, but I can easily picture the angels at Mount Carmel watching the day unfold and gazing at Elijah, thinking, "Lucky! We never get to tell people about the power and the love of our mighty God!" Walther continues: "Without doubt these rescued people will forever and ever thank those by whose ministry they were saved from perdition and brought back into life everlasting. They are, of all people, most despised and even hated by the world. Nevertheless their estate and office is the most glorious of all."[5] Right there lies the unusual and unexpected paradox of ministry: "Most despised and even hated by the world," and at the same time, an office and calling that is "the most glorious of all."

The ten chapters of this book are intended to outline the journey that, in one way or another, we all take, some more successfully than others. We'll look at the lessons we absolutely must learn along the way, lessons about the hazards and pitfalls that, ironically, are the way God teaches us to rely on his grace, just like he taught Elijah, the poster boy for church worker anxiety,

Elijah's unrealized hopes for ministry are not that different from what most of us experience.

burnout and despair. Elijah's unrealized hopes for ministry are not that different from what most of us experience at the end of another long week or month, looking back and wondering what difference our efforts have made.

Most professions involve hard work, but I'm convinced that professional church workers are often blind-sided when they discover the three dangers of a life in ministry: first, that the calling into ministry can actually be hazardous to their own life of faith; second, how often the call to ministry can be destructive to intimate relationships; and third, how the burdens of a career in ministry can ultimately drive a person out of the ministry entirely. Jesus warned his followers that this calling would be both a great blessing and a hardship. "Truly I tell you, no one who has left home or brothers or sisters or mother or father or children or fields for me and the gospel will fail to receive a hundred times as much in this present age: homes, brothers, sisters, mothers, children and fields— along with persecutions—and in the age to come eternal life" (Mark 10:29-30). Somehow, we're still caught off guard, thinking it won't really happen to us.

Take a few moments right now to pause and reflect on your own call into ministry. What was the process of discernment like for you? When did you first sense God was calling you to service in the church? How did he make the call clear and certain for you? Was it a short process or was it a call that was spread out across a number of years? Were others involved in your discernment, or was it a journey you took mostly alone? God calls us from our widely disparate places and situations into lives of ministry, but I do expect that one thing we all shared was a passion and an excitement to get started in ministry as soon as possible. There's no time like the first days of ministry in a Christian congregation for visions of the great blessings that lie in wait in the days ahead. Our idealism and enthusiasm are at their highest level.

The harsh reality of ministry life can threaten the passion for ministry at any point in a long career, but particularly in the early years if we're unprepared for the challenges that lie ahead.

The history of the Christian church is framed around the long story of the struggle and sacrifice of those who followed the call into ministry. Do their sufferings and trials mean that God was not with them, that he was not at work in them and through them? Not at all! What they learned along the way was that it was the hard that made it great. It was in their most challenging times that they looked to the Lord and found him right with them in power and grace. Lesson Two on the journey toward wholeness in ministry reads like this: "Ministry is great, but hard because it's the way of the cross." It's a lesson we need planted deeply in our hearts so that it will carry us through the difficult times we'll be called to endure.

Fortunately, we have good mentors in the prophets, apostles and saints who have gone before us. They all endured because they did fix their eyes on Jesus. Our Lord knew that he would be glorified only through his cross and death (see John 12:23-26). It's in the midst of our own struggles that the glory of Jesus comes to us also, and so, by faith, we keep our eyes fixed on Jesus to find his strength to continue.

THE APOSTLES AND THE WAY OF THE CROSS

The first generation of Christian ministers wrestled with the same paradox of the struggle and the joy that we do. One of my favorite stories of church worker wellness is the response of Paul and Silas to the brutal treatment they received in Philippi, recorded in Acts 16. It always surprises me how casually Luke mentions the torture they endured in the vastly understated little prepositional phrase, "After they had been severely flogged..." and again in his understatement of their suffering as the jailer "put them in the inner cell and fastened their feet in the stocks" (Acts 16:23-24).

These two faithful servants had no desire to sit in the places of honor or to "lord it over" others. Their response to the way of the cross was pure joy. "About midnight Paul and Silas were praying and singing hymns to God..." (Acts 16:25). There was only one force in the universe strong enough to carry them through the unwarranted persecution they endured: the gift of joy, received by faith in a compassionate and ever-present Lord. The cross of Christ had become for them not a theological concept or a mere symbol of God's love. For them it was a way of life. They had fully embodied the life of dying and living a new life in the power of the Spirit. The words they shared flowed out of the transformed lives they had experienced and were experiencing daily. They picked up their crosses and followed where Jesus was leading them.

Paul told his young apprentice Timothy that it's the hard parts of ministry that make it great. Paul invited him to join in the suffering of a life under the cross.

> So do not be ashamed of the testimony about our Lord or of me
> his prisoner. Rather, join with me in suffering for the gospel, by the
> power of God (2 Timothy 1:8).

And Paul told young Timothy, "You then, my son, be strong in the grace that is in Christ Jesus. And the things you have heard me say in the presence of many witnesses entrust to reliable people who will also be qualified to teach others. Join with me in suffering, like a good soldier of Christ Jesus" (2 Timothy 2:1-3).

The way of the cross is a recurring theme in all of the New Testament writers. Consider the following examples from Luke, Peter and the Lord's brother, James. As you read each of the following New Testament texts, consider how there is always a purpose, an ultimate benefit for us and for the

Church because of the struggles we face for one reason and for one reason only: God is working his wonders in us through the challenges we face.

Acts 14:21-22 — "Then they returned to Lystra, Iconium and Antioch, strengthening the disciples and encouraging them to remain true to the faith. 'We must go through many hardships to enter the kingdom of God,' they said."

1 Peter 1:6-7 — "In all this you greatly rejoice, though now for a little while you may have had to suffer grief in all kinds of trials. These have come so that the proven genuineness of your faith—of greater worth than gold, which perishes even though refined by fire—may result in praise, glory and honor when Jesus Christ is revealed."

James 1:2-4 — "Consider it pure joy, my brothers and sisters, whenever you face trials of many kinds, because you know that the testing of your faith produces perseverance. Let perseverance finish its work so that you may be mature and complete, not lacking anything."

I hope that in the midst of the sacrifices you make and the hardships you endure for the sake of your ministry that you are learning Lesson Two on the journey toward wholeness: "...because it's the way of the cross." I hope you find it as encouraging as I do that those who have gone before us in ministry all learned this crucial lesson and have, by the grace of God, endured the crosses that the Lord has allowed them to bear. We're easily blindsided by how hard service in the Church can be. It is hard, and because of our weakness, we don't naturally bear it well. Like Elijah and like Paul, we have those times of frustration, discouragement and even despair, but we're not without hope. We stand in a long line of the faithful before us.

My favorite ancient Collect of the Church is a prayer for the journey. I keep a copy of this prayer in my wallet and I've turned to it many times over the years for comfort and hope in the journey. The ancient cry of God's people goes like this: "Lord God, you have called Your servants to ventures of which we cannot see the ending, by paths as yet untrodden, through perils unknown. Give us faith to go out with courage, not knowing where we go, but only that Your hand is leading us and Your love supporting us; through Jesus Christ our Lord. Amen."[6]

Elijah learned that ministry is great, but hard. Jesus and the Apostles taught us that ministry is the way of the cross. Before we get to more hopeful news, let's explore what we know about the often overwhelming nature of the tasks of parish and school ministry and some of the research on how church workers are bearing up under the load.

NOT FINISHED YET!

Take a few minutes to consider whether Lesson Two, "Ministry is the way of the cross" is a lesson about ministry that you've taken to heart.

» What did you read in this chapter that resonates most deeply? What made you say to yourself, "That's really true!"?

» How would you phrase Lesson Two differently?

» What did Darrell not discuss in this chapter that really could have been mentioned?

» If this is a lesson you've already learned from your own experience, when did you first discover that it was true?

» What needs your further contemplation before moving on to the next chapter?

MINISTRY TEAM CONVERSATION STARTERS FOR LESSON TWO

» Look at the comments from church workers at the beginning of this Lesson. Do any of them resonate with you? Why?

» In what ways have you (and your family!) borne the cross of ministry? How have you struggled emotionally, relationally, physically, financially, spiritually, or vocationally?

» What do you think of Walther's statement that if the angels were capable of envy, "they would unquestionably envy every teacher of the Gospel"?

» Who are some of your models for bearing the crosses of ministry with faith and perseverance?

» Which Scripture promises encourage you through the hard times of ministry?

3

And Overwhelmed Is a Way of Life

ELIJAH CRASHED. It was a precipitous drop from the highest of highs after the Lord's victory on Mount Carmel to the lowest of lows as he panicked in fear and ran for his life. It was a crash; a complete collapse and an abrupt descent from absolute victory to the depths of despair.

Imagine Elijah's sudden despair to discover that God's display of judgment had apparently made no difference in the palace. It was Queen Jezebel (who had not witnessed the miracle on the mountain) and not his "new friend" Ahab who still directed the political and religious forces of the north. In my Bible, it's only about an inch down the page from 1 Kings 18:46, "... he ran ahead of Ahab all the way to Jezreel" to 1 Kings 19:3, "Elijah was afraid and ran for his life." That's a complete reversal, and it's the most puzzling part of the story. How did this mighty prophet of the Lord, who by all appearances was in tremendous condition spiritually, physically and emotionally, experience such a complete and utter collapse?

It would seem that Elijah was not quite as fit as he thought he was. It turns out, as we'll see in this chapter, self-awareness is not always a strength of people in church work professions. Ministry is great, but hard, in part because we make it hard by not tending to our own spiritual, physical, emotional and vocational wellbeing. Since following Jesus in church leadership is the way of the cross, our trust in God's strength, not in our own capacity, is essential.

Why Elijah was more fragile than he may have appeared is a mystery, but there are some hints in the text. If it's true he assumed that the battle on Mount Carmel indicated the end of the war for the hearts of the nation, his assumption was clearly premature. He may also have overestimated his own spiritual maturity. Walther Maier notes that compared to previous episodes in his prophetic career, there was no sustaining Word from God during this critical juncture. "[W]hen he is in great danger (so he thinks), Elijah receives no word from Yahweh as to what he should do. Elijah always before had acted and been directed by a word from God... Now, such a word from Yahweh is absent."[7] And if he was counting on support from Ahab, it wasn't there. So although the protecting and sustaining hand of God would never leave him, Elijah seems convinced that it had. Left to his own limited capacity, he feared for his life, ran into the desert, and collapsed under the broom tree.

Ministry is great, but it's hard, and we're not always as prepared to face the challenges of a life in ministry as we may think we are. This chapter is about the difference between the perception most church workers have of their capacity to endure the hardships of their calling and the harsh reality that most of us are in way over our heads most of the time. Lesson Three on our journey to wellness, "Overwhelmed is a way of life," is intended to pull the rug out from under anyone who thinks they're doing really well most of the time, when in reality we're in jeopardy nearly all of the time.

This chapter comes with a warning label: "Brace yourself. This might hurt a little bit."

After thirty years of making nearly all of the mistakes I'll enumerate throughout this book, I chose to leave the parish ministry that I love so much in order to serve as Program Director of Grace Place Wellness Ministries. It was a tough call, but I did it in order to equip other professional church workers to stay in ministry for long and vibrant careers. My only qualification for my current position is that after three decades of parish ministry, I ended healthier and stronger than I began, in large part due to the privilege of attending the first Grace Place Wellness Retreat with my wife Carol in 2000. My current calling has positioned me to observe others in church work professions, and what I've observed matches my own experience and strongly affirms the research you're about to explore.

While church workers are often unaware of the dangers of a life in ministry, church leaders who are asked to swoop in and help pick up the pieces after a ministry failure know the dangers all too well.

The psychological community started to get indications decades ago that there was something going on with church work professionals. By mid-twentieth century it became widely recognized that a disproportionate number of professional church workers were seeking the aid of mental health professionals. Clergy burnout as a specific mental health disorder became a topic of investigation. I count myself among those who managed the overwhelming load of unreasonable expectations (both the church's and my own) pretty poorly most of the time.

Since those early studies, the research has expanded dramatically. In my own denomination, studies from 1999 and from 2017 showed that we are in most ways no different from church workers of other traditions. Those who supervise people in ministry know there's a problem in the ranks. In 2012, the Office of National Mission of The Lutheran Church Missouri Synod set six mission priorities for the church which included "#5. Nurture pastors, missionaries and professional church workers to promote spiritual, emotional and physical well-being."[8] By 2016, the national convention of our church body had established a floor committee dedicated entirely to the topic of church worker wellbeing. By the 2019 national convention of the LCMS (where delegates wore name badge lanyards imprinted "Church Worker Wellness"), the majority of the thirty-five District Presidents specifically noted in their official reports to the synod that church worker wellness had become one of the top priorities of their middle judicatories. The same pattern is seen in nearly all church bodies in America today. Leaders in the church are beginning to recognize what frontline church workers often fail to see.

STUDY OF CHURCH WORKER JOB RESPONSIBILITIES

The most extensive research we've found on church worker wellness is focused on the specific demands and lifestyles of parish pastors. My thirty years in team ministry working in close partnership with Directors of Christian Education, Deaconesses, church musicians and parochial school teachers tells me that it's a very short leap to extrapolate the research conclusions and apply it to nearly all church work professionals. The conclusions of the research are frightening. The expectations placed on pastors, teachers and parish professionals are nearly unimaginable.[9]

Study after study suggests that because of the breath of different kinds of work required of those who serve in the church and school, church workers are expected to be something like "expert generalists," able to shift gears rapidly, change hats, and utilize completely different skill sets at a moment's notice. Considering how impactful the work we do is in the lives of children and adults, it's no wonder overwhelmed is a way of life for church workers.

Lesson One taught us that ministry is hard. The growing data from research suggests that it's likely harder than any of us expected, and also that none of us are equipped, gifted or trained to perform all of the tasks of ministry up to the expectations of either ourselves or the members of the congregation.

THE HIGHS AND THE LOWS

How are church workers holding up under these extraordinary demands? Here the research suggests that there's something of a paradox at work. Church work professionals tend to report a very high level of satisfaction with their occupational life. They find the work challenging, rewarding and extremely satisfying. On the other hand, research into the levels of stress and the risk for burnout suggest that a significant portion

...like the person standing with one foot in a tub of boiling water and the other in a tub of ice water commenting, "On average, I'm feeling pretty good."

of church workers are in jeopardy of experiencing the kind of crash that Elijah did.[10]

A recent study uses self-reported indicators of wellness such as confidence in their calling, physical and emotional exhaustion, ministry satisfaction and fit with their current ministry to measure the risk for burnout[11] and concludes that most church workers report that they feel they are doing fairly well, but as many as one-third are at risk of burnout. And almost all church workers report that they have direct knowledge of others who left the ministry because of high levels of stress and burnout.[12]

This paradox might indicate the nature of the problem. Professional church workers are quick to recognize the stress of an overwhelmed lifestyle as the cause of a peer's departure from active ministry, but we're not self-aware enough to recognize its effects in our own lives. I hope you are among those who consider yourself to be doing well. There is, however, reason for concern even when we're feeling positive about how we're faring in ministry. It's entirely possible that both sides of this paradox are true. We do love the work that we do and find it tremendously rewarding, but may at the same time be unaware of how severely the demands of ministry are depleting us spiritually, emotionally, relationally and physically. It's sort of like the person standing with one foot in a tub of boiling water and the other in a tub of ice water commenting, "On average, I'm feeling pretty good." A very rewarding career in ministry does not necessarily counterbalance or equalize the impact that the burdens of the calling present.

Pastors, youth ministers, Deaconesses, and Christian school teachers are all intimately involved in the most intensely impassioned moments in the lives of the children and families we serve as well as the most intensely emotional moments of congregational life. We're there for both the celebrating and for the grieving. We're right in the middle of Christmas Eve worship and also right in the middle of the congregational vote to close the school. We celebrate with young people as they confess their faith on Confirmation Day and grieve when we don't see them again until the following Easter. We wouldn't have it any other way, but the emotional tide threatens our wellbeing.

Like Elijah, when we fail to be self-aware enough to recognize the strain of ministry, our wellbeing, and the wellbeing of those we love, is in jeopardy. In our work with ministry professionals at Grace Place Wellness we often see indications of burnout and the inattention of church workers to their own wellbeing. It's rarely a good sign when a church worker ends up on the nightly news. It's usually a sign of poor boundaries caused by inadequate self-care that lead to misbehavior.

Far too many teachers and parish professionals leave church work every year and the number seems to be on the rise. Often when we talk to those who leave church ministry we find that they are unable to identify the contributing causes; it seems that they just reached the point of being unable to continue, without fully understanding the reasons why. That's reason for concern. Our ministry began in the heart of a medical doctor, John Eckrich, who regularly asked his patients who were church workers, married to church workers, or the children of church workers, "How are you doing?" Despite the "glittering image"[13] we are tempted to present to our congregations, that our spiritual, emotional and relational houses are in perfect order, it doesn't fly in the doctor's office when he's looking at pictures of ulcers and lab tests of blood pressure, blood sugar and all variety of stress related illness trending well above the national average.

It's okay to be human, and it's okay to be overwhelmed with the responsibilities of ministry, but it's only okay when we're self-aware enough to take Lesson Three fully to heart: "Overwhelmed is a way of life." Realistic decisions about self-care are grounded in a fully informed awareness of the nature of the task, and for church workers it means coming to grips with our reality: we face a never-ending task for which we are never fully equipped.

FULLY HUMAN, AND FULLY AWARE

The root cause of the church worker wellness epidemic is the tendency for church workers to become what David Tripp calls "self-swindlers." Tripp writes in "Dangerous Calling,"

> If you aren't daily admitting to yourself that you are a mess and
> in daily and rather desperate need for forgiving and transforming
> grace, and if the evidence around has not caused you to abandon

your confidence in your own righteousness, then you are going to give yourself to the work of convincing yourself that you are okay. How do you do that? Well, you point to the ample evidence the fallen world gives you, that the people and situations around you are flawed and broken and are, therefore, the reason you respond to life the way you do. You tell yourself again and again that you are not the problem — that it is or they are, but not you. And you tell yourself that you really don't need to change; it's the people and circumstances around you that need to change.[14]

Without a fully aware self-assessment of how the work of ministry is impacting your life, the wellness journey comes to a halt. We live within a paradox: we love what we do, but what we do can be dangerous to our wellbeing.

We humans, so they say, are the only creatures capable of self-deception, and the research noted above indicates that ministers take full advantage of that deadly capacity. Far too often, we end up like Elijah under the broom tree, thinking to ourselves, "I never saw it coming!"

The irony here is that Jesus came to save sinners, of whom we are the worst. There's not a day when we aren't just as desperately in need of the grace of God as any other of his children. Presenting our glittering image, acting as if we've got it "all together all the time," only compounds the problem. Church workers who try to convince others (and themselves!) that everything is fine put themselves at risk. It's a paradox of our profession that we, who should know this better than most, far too often stumble along seemingly unaware that the gospel of grace we share with others applies fully

> Church workers who try to convince others (and themselves!) that everything is fine put themselves at risk.

to ourselves first! We proclaim the reality of human frailty, but fail to accurately assess our own. Because of the pressure exerted upon us from both the inside and the outside, we the feel the compulsion to present ourselves to the world as superhuman, for some reason not fully subject to the effects of the fallen sinful human nature.

HUMANS MAKE THE BEST CHURCH WORKERS

So how do we bear up under the weight of the cross, the enormity of our calling within the limits of the frailty of our humanity? This may sound counterintuitive, and even a bit bizarre, but overwhelmed church workers are actually good for the advance of the gospel. If you feel overwhelmed a good part of the time in ministry, you're in good company. I believe that you're supposed to feel that way. When we're overwhelmed by the enormity of the task and the unending nature of the harvest field stretching out before us, we become dependent on a power far greater than our own, the strength of God himself working in us and through us.

While it's not my favorite superhero movie, "The Green Lantern" has a few good moments. Hal Jordan (played by Ryan Reynolds) was, of all creatures, a human chosen to wear the ring of the Green Lantern, protector of a vast region of space. He was immediately overwhelmed by his responsibilities, but soon got caught up in the headiness of his new found powers and thought he was pretty great stuff. At the climactic point of the struggle between the forces of good and evil, Hal realized how overmatched he was against the bad guy seeking universal domination, and he almost gave up the battle, but his compassion, considered by other Lanterns a uniquely human weakness, compelled him to keep fighting. After Hal, the most unlikely hero of all, saved the universe from certain doom with the help of a power far greater than his own strength, the movie concludes with my favorite part, the sonorous voice of the narrator offering a closing epilog as the final credits get ready to roll.

"Of all the Lanterns who have ever worn the ring there was one who's light shined brightest. At first his humanity was thought to be a weakness, and yet it proved to be his greatest strength."[15]

I've grown fond of saying, "Humans make the best church workers." Elijah was fully human; maybe more human than he realized. God in his mercy took him aside on the mountaintop retreat at Horeb and gave him a new sense of self-awareness. "At first his humanity was thought to be a weakness, and yet it proved to be his greatest strength." Humanness is a good thing for church workers, as long as we're able to recognize and manage our frailties appropriately, and rely on the power and grace of God for ministry fruitfulness.

Do you remember the account of Paul and Barnabas in Lystra? After a miraculous healing, the crowds worshiped and adored them, but when they heard the shouts of, "The gods have come down to us in human form!" the apostles quickly responded, "Why are you doing this? We too are only men, human like you" (Acts 14:15). That might be a worthy inscription on your classroom or office door: "Your Name Here: Human Like You." Humans make the best church workers because humans like us rely fully on God.

OVERWHELMED AND HUMBLED

Lesson Three, "Overwhelmed is a way of life," sounds bad at first, but with the proper attitude toward our inability to meet every expectation, we just might be better prepared for ministry; overwhelmed, but humbly receptive to God's strength like Moses or Peter. Here are a few of the reasons why "Overwhelmed," if we can come to grips with it, is a good place for us to be.

Overwhelmed makes us receptive to the grace of God in Christ. It's the hammer of God's law that points out how unprepared and incapable of the work of ministry we are; the purpose of the law is to bring us to the point of despair, to confess our unworthiness so that we become open to the rescue that only God can deliver. Grace is amazing only to "a wretch like me."

Overwhelmed confirms our baptismal identity in Christ. Baptism into Christ means baptism into his death. Drowned in flood waters is a perfect picture of being overwhelmed. Facing tasks and responsibilities beyond our capacity keeps us grounded in our reliance on God for everything, reminding us moment by moment through the day who we are and whose we are.

Overwhelmed creates a sense of dependence upon the whole body of Christ and fosters unity and harmony in the church. We'll explore this more in the next chapter. No single part of the body can do it all; each is dependent on the wide variety and diversity of all the others (see 1 Corinthians 12 and Romans 12).

And overwhelmed is humiliating, that is to say, humbling, and it makes us available for God's call. Like Abraham, Moses, Esther, Peter and so many of the Lord's servants who've gone before us, when called, we respond, "God, you've got the wrong person!" The Lord of the church operates today the way he always has, seeking the overwhelmed, because he knows the overwhelmed stay dependent upon him and his strength.

> **And overwhelmed is humiliating, that is to say, humbling, and it makes us available for ministry.**

Humans make the best church workers and overwhelmed humans are in the best position to serve in the strength of God. In order to manage "Overwhelmed as a Way of Life," we must find a way to face the reality that as long as we pursue ministry, the pervasive sense of being overwhelmed will be with us, mentally, relationally, physically and spiritually. It means having not just a solid theology of who God is, but a firm and realistically grounded anthropology, an understanding who I am. Gary Harbaugh suggests, "We are called not away from our humanness, but through that humanness to God. The incarnation of Christ frees us to be fully human. Only by being who and what I am can I adequately respond as a whole person to the (w)holistic reaction which is stress."[16]

Fortunately, we're not called into this work alone. Well before God ever called us to tend his little lambs, he called us to be members of the flock. It's in our membership in the body of Christ that we can find a great source of God's sustaining grace for ministry.

_____

NOT FINISHED YET!

Take a few minutes to consider whether Lesson Three, "Overwhelmed is a way of life" is a lesson about ministry that you've taken to heart.

» What did you read in this chapter that resonates most deeply? What made you say to yourself, "That's really true!"?

» How would you phrase Lesson Three differently?

» What did Darrell not discuss in this chapter that really could have been mentioned?

» If this is a lesson you've already learned from your own experience, when did you first discover that it was true?

» What needs your further contemplation before moving on to the next chapter?

MINISTRY TEAM CONVERSATION STARTERS FOR LESSON THREE

» What do you think has motivated the recent emphasis on church worker wellness by denominational and regional church leadership?

» What examples can you give of the unrealistic expectations placed on church work professionals? Why does this happen? How does your ministry team (Pastor and staff; Principal and faculty) work together to manage the unrealistic expectations?

» In what ways have you seen that overwhelmed is a way of life in ministry? How do the love of ministry and the strength of Christ counterbalance it?

» How have you experienced the paradox of a love of ministry and the overwhelming demands?

» Read 1 Corinthians 3:5-9. What does it mean to rely on God's strength to do ministry?

» Why do humans make the best church workers?

4

So Don't Try This Alone

IF IT'S TRUE THAT MINISTRY IS both a joyful adventure and a journey of hardship, then the beginning lessons on the journey to wellness read, "Ministry is great, but hard because it's the way of the cross and overwhelmed is a way of life." Lesson Four follows right behind with a word of promise and blessing: "... so don't try this alone."

When the nation of Israel was at its best, the leaders and their people were of one heart and mind in worship, service and mutual care and compassion. It's the same today in the Christian church. Church workers need the unconditional love and support of their families to be at their best. Team ministry marked by mutual trust and respect, led by the Spirit, bearing fruit in Christ's name, can be a beautiful representation of the body of Christ in action. Church workers and congregations need each other to strive forward in mission and ministry, so Lesson Four says, "Don't try this alone."

In the most heartbreaking cry that came out of Elijah's lips while on his mountaintop retreat, he called out in misery, "I am the only one left"

(1 Kings 19:10). To his clouded way of thinking, the burden of bringing the nation back to obedience had fallen squarely upon his shoulders and the burden of it was too much for him. Don't try this alone? Elijah came face to face with the harsh reality that he couldn't do this alone. He collapsed in despair, all alone, with neither the strength nor the passion to continue. Ministry is an isolating profession, and Elijah quickly discovered that this prophet business was no job to try on your own. Even Han Solo didn't fly solo!

So who are we flying with? First and foremost, we take the journey of ministry with our families. We'll dig deeper into the stress of life on a ministry family in Lesson Seven, but a few thoughts are called for here. Church workers tend to be married at a rate higher than the national average, and our families are always impacted by our lives in ministry. We don't know anything about Elijah's family. They are not key players in the unfolding drama. There is only one reference in 1 Kings 19 to Elijah's family. His ancestors were presumably faithful followers of Yahweh who had previously finished their course on earth. At his moment of collapse, when he fell exhausted under the broom tree, the burdens of ministry had become so overwhelming that his last desire was to breathe his final breath and be with those who had already died. "'I have had enough, Lord,' he said. 'Take my life; I am no better than my ancestors" (1 Kings 19:4). For all we know, Elijah is an example of the vulnerability of single church workers because of the stress of separation from networks of familial support.

It's also true that church worker spouses and children endure many of the anxieties of church work right along with the called worker. Families manage the stresses of ministry life in a wide variety of different ways, but the key is the establishment of good patterns of communication, gracious forgiveness and family unity. Each of these topics will be pursued in more detail later, but Lesson Four, "So don't try this alone," shows why a strong family life is so important.

We take the journey of church work also with the people we serve in the congregation; the church and the school. Congregational care and support for church workers often happens more naturally for pastors and the churches they serve than it does for other school and parish church professionals. The Pastor is the most public figure, and often the only called worker. Church members know the Pastor and his family members by name and are responsive to their needs. Their salaries, vacation allowances, and other forms of support are typically much more significant than that of other workers. When it comes to support and encouragement, the non-ordained workers in the church often experience inequities, feeling like "stagehands" in the church's ministry production, as a deaconess friend of mine put it. "So don't try this alone" encourages us to pursue close bonds of nurture and care with the congregation and its leaders.

And we take the journey on a very intimate level with our partners in ministry, our fellow called workers. For parish professionals in church and school, the most significant encouragement they receive is that which they offer to one another. That's why healthy team ministry is an essential component of a life in Christian service marked by joy. Churches have a biblical responsibility to care for their called staff, but it takes a long time for churches, if they haven't been supportive, to learn how. There's no reason why partners in team ministry shouldn't be working on the practices of mutual care every day.

In God's design for his kingdom's laborers, all ministry is team ministry. Elijah's ministry got off to a great start, and even though the nation was enduring a difficult time, he threw himself into his calling with the passion and the joy of knowing that he was God's chosen prophet for his time and place. Elijah, however, was deserted by the nation's leadership. In God's design for Israel, the prophets, priests and kings would all represent the Lord to the people with one united, purposeful and passionate voice. At precisely the time when Elijah could have used some support, King Ahab and Queen Jezebel turned on him and became his worst enemies. Not only did they not have his back, they were the ones who threatened him with annihilation!

THE DREAM AND THE REALITY OF TEAMS

A positive sense of community, uplifting and encouraging relationships with co-workers, is critically important in the workplace. Everyone wants to feel that the work they do is significant, that it makes the world a better place, and everyone needs to have a sense of competence in their assigned tasks, but even if you're convinced that you're making a difference in the world, and that you have the skills to get the job done, if you don't get along with the people on your team, and if you do not share a significant amount of trust and mutual respect, you'll be highly unlikely to thrive in your job or stay committed to it for the long haul.

Legendary basketball coach John Wooden once said, "It takes ten hands to make a basket." When the team is playing together, striving together as a unified whole for a common objective, the work becomes play and the smiles and shouts of joy drown out every opposing force. When one player is feeling left alone to carry the burden of winning the game, the joy departs.

> John Wooden once said, "It takes ten hands to make a basket."

When I think of teamwork, I think of church workers. When unity in the church prevails, church workers flourish. When unity suffers, it sounds too much like Elijah's story in 1 Kings 19 and, sadly, like the story of many called workers and their places of service.

The primary responsibility for unity in team ministry lies with the lead pastor of the congregation, even where there is a school administrator responsible for building a faculty team. Unity in a church staff is enhanced when a common vision is shared, when all members of the staff feel that their contributions to the vision are appreciated, and when reasonable expectations of each member are established. Teachers, Directors of Christian Education, Deaconesses and most every category of church workers are specifically trained in the dynamics of team ministry. That's rarely true of pastors.

The challenge for many lead pastors is that they were not trained to support, bless, and create an environment of opportunity and significance for others in team ministry. Most congregations in America are served by one called professional church worker: the Pastor. Most pastors learned the ropes of ministry life in those settings. By the time they are called to lead a team of others, the seminary course on Team Ministry may be long forgotten. But the benefits of building a unified team of ministers to lead the congregation can hardly be overstated.

My introduction to team ministry was less than ideal.

In our denomination, the seminary and District Presidents work together to place graduates in their first church. I was asked by the placement committee how I would respond to "a very stressful team ministry situation." I found it curious that none of my classmates remembered being asked that question. My curiosity was satisfied a few years later when I discovered the church where I had been placed had been served by eight Assistant Pastors in the previous sixteen years. I learned that my immediate predecessor left the ministry entirely after less than two years. A son of the Senior Pastor, a church work professional himself, would pull me aside when in town for a visit and ask how I was doing. "I know my dad can be kind of hard on the assistants." After five years, one of the neighboring pastors suggested to me, "That's some kind of a record, isn't it?" I stayed more than five years until the Pastor announced his retirement. I learned a lot along the way.

I learned even more as an Associate at my next church. The Pastor there had built a wonderful climate of trust, openness and respect. It was a large, growing church where ministry was great, but hard, and overwhelmed was a way of life, but none of us on the team ever felt that we were in it alone. Sometimes when discussing our particular assignments in ministry and the decisions we had made, our leader told us he thought we were nuts, but that he would support us one hundred percent. Sometimes he asked our opinions on difficult choices he had to make. Even if we disagreed with his direction, we told him, "Outside the doors of this office, no one will ever know we disagree. We will speak with one voice to the congregation." The hardest part of accepting a call to serve as a sole pastor in a different state was saying farewell to my partners in team ministry at that church.

And the unity we shared as leaders in ministry impacted the life of the entire congregation.

DESIGNED FOR UNITY

"All the believers were one in heart and mind" (Acts 4:32). Can you remember your first hint that not all was love and concord at Concordia Church? Or that peace was often missing from Peace Church or that the members of St. Peter's, St. Paul's or St. John's did not always behave so saintly? Disunity, division into interest groups and hostility between called workers and people, has plagued the Christian Church since the days of St. Paul's letters to conflicted congregations, but that is not the Lord's intention; we were called and gathered for unity.

Unity is the driving theme of the Letter to the Ephesians where Paul describes the mystery of God's will, "to bring all things in heaven and on earth together under one head, even Christ" (Ephesians 1:10). The historic cultural and religious division between Jews and Gentiles was the critical issue of church unity in Paul's day and chapter two of Ephesians describes how God has removed all barriers by the cross. In the churches of our time, it's often the division between called church workers and members that paralyzes the work of ministry. Consider the bonds of a congregation's workers and its members as you read these familiar words: "For he himself is our peace, who has made the two groups one and has destroyed the barrier, the dividing wall of hostility, by setting aside in his flesh the law with its commands and regulations. His purpose was to create in himself one new humanity out of the two, thus making peace, and in one body to reconcile both of them to God through the cross, by which he put to death their hostility" (Ephesians 2:14-16). When our focus is on the uniting power of the gospel of Christ, the Lord himself is at work in our midst to bring concord to Concordia and peace to Peace congregation, and to help the saints at St. Peter's, St. Paul's and St. John's to behave and serve together in ways that proclaim the work of Christ.

Lesson One tells us that "Ministry is great, but hard..." and Lesson Four tempers the hardness of ministry by adding, "...so don't try this alone." In the service of installation for professional church workers, the congregation is specifically invited to be a blessing to those whom they have called to serve them and to serve with them in the ministry of the church and school. In fact, the congregation is called upon in the rite of installation to vow before God, before the called workers, and before one another that they will indeed, with the help of God, pray for, encourage and support their workers and their families in every way necessary for them to thrive in the work of ministry. That's in keeping with Paul's own personal intention for his relationship with the congregations he served.

SUPPORT AND ACCOUNTABILITY

At Grace Place Wellness Ministries we strongly encourage congregational Church Worker Support Committees as a way to help churches create an environment where their called workers can flourish in ministry.

A Church Worker Support Committee is formed for the purpose of building trust and openness between the called workers of the congregation and its leaders so that they can gather regularly and ask the questions, "What's it like to be in ministry here?" and "What can we do to make this a better environment for our church and school employees so that they are thriving in their roles?" When the church's workers are at their best, spiritually, relationally, financially, emotionally and physically, the congregation benefits from their vitality, peace and joy. When church workers are struggling, everyone, the church workers, their families, and the whole congregation suffers.

The intention of the committee is to build trust to the degree that the church workers can speak the truth with love and bring up the issues that hinder effective ministry, such as gossip, unrealistic expectations, inadequate remuneration and benefits, etc. It often takes a great deal of time to build that level of trust and respect. It's not necessary that Elders, School Board, or Church Council members serve on the committee, but there should be an appropriate, confidential reporting procedure to the governance groups so that concerns can be addressed. When a church operates a parochial school as part of their ministry, a separate committee sensitive to the unique requirements of teachers and staff to flourish should be established.

MUTUALLY ENCOURAGED

There are some beautiful passages in the first chapter of Romans, but the one I love even more than verse sixteen, "For I am not ashamed of the gospel..." is the little unnoticed paragraph that falls in the forgotten space right before. Paul writes, "I long to see you so that I may impart to you some spiritual gift to make you strong— that is, that you and I may be mutually encouraged by each other's faith" (Romans 1:11-12, emphasis added). Wow, that's a powerful description of the church and its workers! Did you notice both parts? First, typical for a church worker, Paul said that he wanted to impart to the Roman church a spiritual blessing, but it's the second part that churches and their called workers need to hear and remember. The Apostle also wanted to receive a blessing from the church. In the unity that they shared, bound together by the ligaments that the Holy Spirit provides, they would each be a blessing to the other, minister blessing people and people blessing all of the ministers of the church, ordained and non-ordained, and their families. Support and accountability can help make that happen.

Pastor Doug Dommer recently retired after 38 years of ministry in the same congregation, Salem Lutheran in Tomball, Texas. In his farewell sermon he succinctly described the difference between those congregations that understand the importance of mutual trust, respect and love between a congregation's workers and people and those who don't. He said, "Many churches eat their pastors alive. Salem loves their pastors to death."[17] I'm convinced that the reason this pastor and congregation survived their many trials together and more importantly, joined together in dynamic gospel witness to their community for so many years was because Pastor Dommer and the church he served learned this important lesson early on: "Don't try this alone."

At the conclusion of Elijah's time on retreat he went back into prophetic ministry in the kingdom, but he didn't go alone. God gave him a promise and a command. The promise? "I reserve seven thousand in Israel − all whose knees have not bowed down to Baal" (1 Kings 19:18). The command? "Anoint Elisha son of Shaphat from Abel Meholah to succeed you as prophet" (1 Kings 19:16). We need partners in ministry and communities of the faithful just as God gave Elijah a prophetic partner and surrounded him with a nation of faithful support. It was the Lord's way of telling the prophet, "Don't try this alone."

I was always at my best when team ministry, family, and congregational partnerships were strong. Mutual encouragement of the kind Paul spoke of was always a great source of joy, the kind that can carry a struggling church worker through difficult times. But what, exactly, is the joy of the Lord? To that question we now turn in Lesson Five.

NOT FINISHED YET!

Take a few minutes to consider whether Lesson Four, "So don't try this alone" is a lesson about ministry that you've taken to heart.

» What did you read in this chapter that resonates most deeply? What made you say to yourself, "That's really true!"?

» How would you phrase Lesson Four differently?

» What did Darrell not discuss in this chapter that really could have been mentioned?

» If this is a lesson you've already learned from your own experience, when did you first discover that it was true?

» What needs your further contemplation before moving on to the next chapter?

MINISTRY TEAM CONVERSATION STARTERS FOR LESSON FOUR

(After Lesson Seven you'll have a chance to explore these themes more extensively. Lay the groundwork for that conversation by discussing the following questions.)

» In what ways have you experienced encouragement for your ministry from your parents, spouse, and children?

» When did you first learn the difference that a strong, unified team ministry can make in your wellbeing? In what ways does your supervisor (Pastor; Principal) make you feel empowered for ministry?

» Share an example of a church you know that really understands how to support its workers. Share an example of one that doesn't. What makes the difference?

» Who would you like to see serve on a Church Worker Support Committee from your church/school?

5

LESSON FIVE

Joy Fuels Ministry

I PICTURE GOD'S GIFT OF JOY a bit like I remember the opening credits of "Disney's Wonderful World of Color." When Tinkerbell showed up on the screen with a sweep of her wand, everything exploded into bursts of bright, beautiful, cascading color. Since the fruit of the Spirit is joy, wherever he shows up and works his wonders of faith and new life, bursts of joy transform his children's dark gray worlds into rainbows of peace and hope.

Elijah had experienced the joy of the Lord throughout the three year drought: the daily miracle of life-sustaining bread, a child raised from death. Joy sustains us in times of trial. It's evidence that God is still God, working wonders of faith wherever he shows up.

That makes me wonder how Elijah could lose the joy of Mount Carmel so quickly.

It certainly wasn't because God was no longer at work. Elijah had prayed, "O Lord, God of Abraham, Isaac and Israel, let it be known today that you are God in Israel," (1 Kings 18:36) and he was indeed still God in Israel. Of that there could be no doubt. Elijah did not lose his joy because God was God; he lost it because Elijah was Elijah. In his human frailty, Elijah had begun to doubt God and his purpose.

Elijah's patience seems to have run out, and doubt crept in. "Thy kingdom come, Thy will be done" had started to evolve into, "Thy kingdom come, MY will be done. NOW!" Luther reminds us that God's kingdom comes and his will is done without our prayers or any of our efforts. The eyes of faith allow us to see the work of the Holy Spirit even while faithless Jezebels rant and rave against it. The blindness of doubt, (to which we are all prone), fails to see God's handiwork. That's when joy departs.

My favorite part of Elijah's retreat is when the Lord spoke to Elijah words of renewal and forgiveness. It resonates across the centuries in the words Jesus spoke by the seashore when the Risen Savior restored Peter who had denied him three times: "Take care of my sheep" (John 21:16). There on the mountain the Lord said to Elijah, "Go back the way you came" (1 Kings 19:15). The fallen prophet was back in business.

After his episode of doubt and despair, Elijah might have been anticipating a harsh word of rebuke from the Lord. Instead he heard, "Go back the way you came. I'm not finished. Neither are you."

The Lord reestablished him in his true identity with a simple word of grace. He was not a miracle worker, just a simple servant of the Word. Can you imagine Peter's joy on the seashore? Or Elijah's on the mountaintop? Maybe not cartwheels, but more like the quiet peace that comes from knowing that God is still God and that he loves me and has plans for my continued service in the kingdom.

I hate to be the one to break the news to you, but it's somewhat unlikely that your ministry exploits will be spoken of in Sunday School classrooms three thousand years from now. I'm glad, however, to let you know that no matter what you're enduring in ministry right now, God is still God; he loves you and he has plans for your continued service in his kingdom.

Lesson Five continues where we left off. "Ministry is great, but hard, because ministry is the way of the cross and overwhelmed is a way of life, but joy is fuel for ministry."

Through the years of my service as Program Director for Grace Place Wellness, I've had the opportunity to ask thousands of church workers, "How are you doing?" After the initial pleasantries and chit-chat, I'll share a little bit about our ministry and then look for the opportunity to ask once again, "But seriously, how are you doing?" As I listen carefully to the response, I'm looking to hear some indication of the joy that fuels ministry, some clue that this beloved, gifted, called and sent minister of the gospel has had on a regular, consistent basis, (and frequently still has,) the faith perspective to step back, to look around and say, "Wow! Jesus did that! That's why I got into this business."

I am shocked by how many church workers have lost the joy of ministry. I'm heartbroken over it, because I'm convinced that joy in ministry is the number one indicator of wellness in the life of a church worker. I've heard far too many church workers tell me that they are only putting in time waiting for the day of their retirement; some even telling me the thought of retirement was the only thing that still brought them joy. I've heard too many church workers speak disparagingly about the members of their flock as if the thought of the people they are called to serve brings them only bitterness and sorrow. I've heard way too many church workers tell stories of years upon years in ministry that were periods of darkness and pain, absent the gift of joy. Those stories sadden me so greatly because the Spirit's gift of joy can carry us through all kinds of setbacks, troubles, and anxieties. In the midst of the struggles for the gospel, regular reminders that God is at work

> I'm convinced that joy in ministry is the number one indicator of wellness.

in us and through us is the greatest encouragement to continue on.

The Lord Jesus has a way of making his presence known by the outpouring of his Holy Spirit in precisely the times we need him most. That's what the theology of the cross teaches: when we are bearing the cross of the calling to serve the One who bore the cross for us, he is revealed to us in all of his power and glory. And in those times when we need him most, those long months of ministry drought when there seems precious little to celebrate, he supplies his gifts, the jars of flour and jugs of oil, the graces that are exactly what we need to persevere. When the dead in sin are raised to life in Christ, when the despairing and discouraged are given new hope, when the broken are healed and restored, it's a sure sign that Jesus has appeared.

When Jesus makes his appearance among his people, he brings gifts. Among the gifts that he gives to his faithful disciples is the gift I pray for you, the gift of joy.

MADE FOR JOY

We were made for joy. When everything is as it should be, when we get those precious glimpses of the Shalom for which we were created, we become aware that we are people designed for a joy that starts deep inside and permeates every part of our being. The natural, original state of humanity in the Garden of Eden was joy, and joy unending will be our inheritance in heaven. Even in this broken life after the Fall, lived in between Eden and Eternity, we get little glimpses of the joy that makes us say, "Now that's what I'm talking about! Life was made for moments like this!"

Joy is critically important for the wellbeing of church workers because it's the antidote for the poison of all that can go wrong in a world broken by sin. The gift of even a few of those moments at the oasis of joy can replenish a spirit that is parched by the trials of life in the wilderness, just as the Spirit of God lifted Paul and Silas into songs of praise after their brutal beating and confinement in the Philippian jail, and just as he lifted Elijah up and sent him back into ministry.

Christian joy transcends the fleeting happiness of a home run, an ice cream cone or a birthday present. Joy gives us glimpses of something greater, something far more wonderful than a sweet treat or a new toy. Joy comes from an encounter with the eternal, with something perfect and pure and incorruptible. And joy can make its appearance even in times when the circumstances of life are lined up poorly.

It's fair to ask "What is Christian joy and where does it come from?" It's certainly an emotion. It's a feeling. I'm sorry if you have an aversion to the emotional side of life, but there's no way around it. Created in the image of an emotional God who feels the full extent and the whole range of emotion, we were made for feelings. It's part of being human. There's certainly danger in living only off of emotion, riding the rollercoaster of highs and lows. Thanks be to God, our salvation is not rooted in how we happen to feel at any given time. The forgiveness of sins, new life under the loving rule of God and our hope for the kingdom that never ends are not dependent on how we may or may not feel at any given moment, but that doesn't change the fact that our emotional life is part of who we are. We're feeling beings because our Father in heaven is an emotional God.

So we ought never forget that in the midst of the whole wide range of negative emotions, joy is still our inheritance. When we share the good news of Christ and are privileged to see the Holy Spirit at work in our humble offerings of service, the proper response is joy. God wants joy to be a constant companion in life, but a surprising and mysterious companion. We should never fall into the trap of thinking that the way of the cross is only a way of suffering and trial. Frederick Buechner warns us,

> We tend to think that joy is not only nor properly religious but
> that it is even the opposite of religion. We tend to think that religion

is sitting stiff and antiseptic and a little bored and that joy is laughter and freedom and reaching out our arms to embrace the whole wide and preposterous earth which is so beautiful that sometimes it nearly breaks our hearts. We need to be reminded that at its heart Christianity is joy and that laughter and freedom and the reaching out of arms are the essence of it.[18]

As children of the living, rejoicing Father, joy is our inheritance, and it's our Father's intention that we live in his joy, to one degree or another, every day of our lives.

Buechner has two additional insights.

One is that joy is all-encompassing; there is nothing of us left over to hate with or to be afraid with, to feel guilty with or to be selfish about. Joy is where the whole thing is poured in one direction, and it is something that by its nature a man never hoards but always wants to share. The second thing is that joy is a mystery because it can happen anywhere, anytime, even under the most unpromising circumstances, even in the midst of suffering, with tears in its eyes. Even nailed to a tree.

What Jesus is saying is that men are made for joy and that anyone who is truly joyous has a right to say that he is doing God's will on this earth. Where you have known joy, you have known him.[19]

Joy is our heritage and a gift from God, but can we pin down a more precise definition of this mysterious thing called joy in order to keep our fuel tanks filled with daily reasons to rejoice?

"A GOOD FEELING IN THE SOUL"

In recent years, I've examined dozens of studies of this gift of the Spirit called joy. The most helpful and satisfying description of Christian joy I've found so far comes from pastor and author John Piper. In a Bible study series on joy, he presents this definition:

> "Christian joy
>
> is a good feeling in the soul,
>
> produced by the Holy Spirit,
>
> as he causes us to see
>
> the beauty of Christ
>
> in the word and in the world."[20]

Before you move on and hear what I like about Piper's definition, take a timeout here for a moment and reflect on what you just read. What do you like about this definition of joy? What word or phrase rings true for you? What leaves you wondering? Does this definition bring a little more clarity to a mysterious topic? What is your experience of joy, and how well does it match up with what Piper describes?

Most of the definitions of joy that I looked at were too technical and theological, almost clinical, and they left me flat, but when I saw this one I was impressed by how thoughtfully Piper had considered the topic of joy and how well he had expressed such a slippery and hard to define concept in simple, clear language. Here are some of the things I like about Piper's definition of Christian joy.

"Christian joy..." It's better than Super Bowl joy. He's talking about the fruit of the Spirit that the saints before us enjoyed, given to you by God himself (Galatians 5:22). Christian joy is intimately connected to the gospel of salvation in Jesus Christ. It is the exclusive treasure of those called to faith. Joy is fuel for ministry because it flows from the good news of the gospel of Christ.

> Joy is fuel for ministry because it flows from the good news of the gospel of Christ.

"...is a good feeling..." That seems understated, but joy comes in a variety of flavors and intensities. It can be overwhelming and rapturous like a roaring waterfall, but it can also be quiet and calm, like a babbling brook. There is a place for the brain and rational thought and reason in our faith, but joy is real. We run on emotion much of the time and joy is fuel for ministry because it's a foundational emotion of life in Christ.

"...in the soul..." It's deep. Joy penetrates the most intimate parts of who we are as children of the heavenly Father. Joy is fuel for ministry because even though the flesh is weak, a heart and will filled with joy continues in the challenging daily tasks of ministry despite forces that would drive us under the broom tree.

"...that is produced by the Holy Spirit..." I love how Piper's definition of joy is grounded in the person and fruit of God the Holy Spirit. It reminds us that our efforts at finding joy will be fruitless (pardon the pun), because joy is a gift that only God can give. Joy is his to give and he loves to give it. Joy is fuel for ministry because all ministry is the work of the Holy Spirit and as he calls us into his harvest fields he also supplies what we need to follow where he is leading.

"...as he causes us to see..." Joy comes from faith. I like the passive phrase "causes us to see" because it gives credit to the Holy Spirit for interrupting our joyless condition. Like someone who grabs your head and turns it so you can see the passing dolphins or the brilliant sunset, it's the work of the Holy Spirit alone to break into our blindness and despair and give joy as a healing, enlightening gift. Joy is fuel for ministry because just when we feel like giving up, he opens the eyes of our hearts to see the work of Jesus.

"...the beauty of Christ..." This is a great expression and the heart of Piper's definition of joy. True joy is grounded in the person and work of Jesus Christ. It's always about Jesus. This world offers what is frail and fleeting and cannot sustain a good feeling in the soul. Jesus can. He is what's beautiful.

When Jesus works his wonders, they are wonders beyond anything else that ever has or ever could happen to us. Beauty brings joy and the perfect beauty of Jesus brings perfect joy, as John the Baptist once said, "The bride belongs to the bridegroom. The friend who attends the bridegroom waits and listens for him, and is full of joy when he hears the bridegroom's voice. That joy is mine and is now complete" (John 3:29). Joy fuels ministry, because we are friends of the Bridegroom.

"...in the word and in the world." First, the Word. Every time we open the scriptures, Jesus is on display. His law condemns me for my sin; his gospel frees me from my desperate need. Always it's the living Jesus who's at work on every page of the Bible doing beautiful things, from creation until his final appearance. The Bible is the story of God's presence among his people. It's a Book of Joy from beginning to end. Joy fuels ministry because the Word of God fuels ministry, and there's always joy in the Word of God.

And since it's a story that is not yet complete, Jesus continues to make himself known in the world around us as he changes peoples' lives by the gospel. When the Spirit opens the eyes of our hearts to see the wondrous working of our Savior in the lives of his faithful people, as he did throughout the history of his children recorded in the Bible, it's cause for a good feeling in the soul. It's a reason for joy. No wonder the angels are jealous! Christian joy is fuel for ministry because the call into ministry is the privilege of being instruments of the only One who can do such wonders of power and love in the lives of his people, and an indicator of a healthy, balanced life in ministry.

There's an old joke that for some Christians, every day is Lent. I will admit that the sentiment is partially correct. Luther once wrote that the washing of Holy Baptism "indicates that the Old Adam in us should by daily contrition and repentance be drowned and die with all sins and evil desires,"[21] but that's only half the story. Christians are gospel people, resurrection people! For believers in Christ, every day is Easter Sunday. Luther continues that baptism also indicates, "that a new man should daily emerge and arise to live before God in righteousness and purity forever."[22] That's joy! No matter what has happened, no matter what I've done or what others have done to me, baptismal renewal is a new birth, a new beginning, the promise of forgiveness, life and salvation, and a reason for rejoicing.

Our denominational President recently wrote, "For the longest time I regarded the texts about joy as mere Law or command. A serious evaluation of these texts has completely changed my mind. When the Gospel is proclaimed with an invitation or even a command to believe the Gospel, the Gospel creates and gives the very thing it demands."[23] Grace and joy, like the pedals on a bicycle, fuel one another, and joy fuels ministry.

JOY AND GRACE

The essence of church worker wellness is to be consciously and continually aware that the joy we proclaim must be first of all the joy we have received by grace. It's the reason Paul and Silas could sing in the Philippian jail after being cursed, beaten and chained. It's the reason that God was able to send the broken and then restored Elijah back the way he came to continue on in his ministry. I'll suggest that for church workers joy is delivered as a gift of grace in three ways every day. First, the joy of the Lord comes to us in our daily walk of faith, living in the grace of God by the Word and the Sacraments. Second, the joy of the Lord comes in the experience of unity in the body of Christ, where love and forgiveness are freely shared. And third, the joy of the Lord comes to us as we humbly share the great good news of God's grace and joy through the work

"Grace Place Wellness nurtures vitality and joy in ministry by inspiring and equipping church workers to lead healthy lives."

of ministry. There is joy in Life with God, Life in Christian Community and Life in Ministry.

The gift of joy in ministry for God's kingdom workers has been the driving force behind the ministry of Grace Place Wellness for years. It defines our mission: "Grace Place Wellness nurtures vitality and joy in ministry by inspiring and equipping church workers to lead healthy lives." The heartbreak of the worker wellness crisis is that so many church workers have seen the joy depart from one, two or all three of those fountains of joy. In the next three chapters, we're going to examine why and how ministers of the gospel are in danger of losing their fuel for ministry, the joy of the Lord. It's going to be a disturbing read for you, so enter into the next part of this book with these gospel promises.

"The apostles left the Sanhedrin, rejoicing because they had been counted worthy of suffering disgrace for the Name. Day after day, in the temple courts and from house to house, they never stopped teaching and proclaiming the good news that Jesus is the Messiah" (Acts 5:41-42).

"May the God of hope fill you with all joy and peace as you trust in him, so that you may overflow with hope by the power of the Holy Spirit" (Romans 15:13).

"Do not grieve, for the joy of the Lord is your strength" (Nehemiah 8:10).

And long, productive, joyful careers in ministry are built upon the foundation of learning these lessons well: Ministry is great but hard, so don't try this alone because ministry is the way of the cross and overwhelmed is a way of life, but joy is fuel for ministry.

Now it's time to take a closer look at those leaky fuel tanks of ours in order to help you get a handle on the dangers that a life in ministry poses to the joy of Life with God, to the joy of Life in Community and the joy of Life in Ministry.

NOT FINISHED YET!

Take a few minutes to consider whether Lesson Five, "Joy is fuel for ministry" is a lesson about ministry that you've taken to heart.

» What did you read in this chapter that resonates most deeply? What made you say to yourself, "That's really true!"?

» How would you phrase Lesson Five differently?

» What did Darrell not discuss in this chapter that really could have been mentioned?

» If this is a lesson you've already learned from your own experience, when did you first discover that it was true?

» What needs your further contemplation before moving on to the next chapter?

MINISTRY TEAM CONVERSATION STARTERS FOR LESSON FIVE

» What brings you the greatest joy in ministry?

» Share why you agree or disagree that "Joy is fuel for ministry"?

» What do you like about John Piper's definition of Christian joy? What needs clarification?

» Who on your ministry team seem to be experiencing the joy of the Lord regularly?

» What takes the joy out of ministry? How does Jesus help you reclaim the joy?

6

LESSON SIX

But Ministry Threatens the Joy of Life with God

IMAGINE THE JOY THE DISCIPLES FELT AT WITNESSING THE MIRACLES OF JESUS. "God did that!" always brings joy. Years after Matthew, Peter and James were gone, John wrote, "That which was from the beginning, which we have heard, which we have seen with our eyes, which we have looked at and our hands have touched — this we proclaim concerning the Word of life... We write this to make our joy complete" (1 John 1:1, 4). Some manuscripts read "... to make your joy complete," and it's understandable that a scribe would conclude that the apostles' joy was something they wanted to share, but John called the joy his very own heritage from the Lord!

I can imagine that John was already thinking of you when he recorded the counsel of Jesus, "Remain in me, and I will remain in you. No branch can bear fruit by itself; it must remain in the vine. Neither can you bear fruit unless you remain in me" (John 15:4). In their ministry internships with the Lord

Jesus, the disciples learned never to try ministry alone. Ministry was shared in teams, and only with the blessing and the presence of Jesus. Earlier, Lesson Four told us "Don't try this alone," affirming that the call into ministry is from the body of Christ, is for the body of Christ and is conducted in the midst of the prayers, encouragement and support of the body of Christ. "Don't try this alone" could also be interpreted to say, "Don't try this alone without the presence and power of God." Lesson Six teaches that people in ministry are in danger of failing to remain in Christ, because, ironically, the call into ministry itself can be a hazard to our intimacy with our Lord. The last Lesson said that "Joy fuels ministry," and this lesson qualifies that truth with the caveat, "... but ministry threatens the joy of life with God." It's a tragic irony, but a harsh reality of ministry, that the call to pick up the mantle of Christian ministry can actually be a hindrance to a vibrant and empowering life with God. This chapter will help unpack the nature of this hazard that has sidetracked so many professional church workers through the centuries.

We're all in constant danger of cracking and leaking joy.

Like Elijah under the broom tree, we're all in constant danger of cracking and leaking joy. We're all so vulnerable because we share in the same broken human condition.

At our best, we're not spiritually healthy. Spiritual wholeness is not our natural condition. If God's Shalom is defined as the gift of everything in life coming together into a beautiful whole, we're more shallow than we are Shalom. The reality of this human life is that we're fractured. We're fashioned by our Creator to be vessels of spiritual joy, to abide in him and to live tuned in to the beauty of Christ at work in us and around us, but we leak, like the jars of clay that we are. Most church workers are leaking in more ways than they recognize.

People can rarely tell when they have bad breath; we're pretty lousy at self-awareness. We might be in serious trouble relationally, emotionally, physically or spiritually and yet be in complete denial. We might be deeply wounded with the joy of ministry puddling around our feet and still bravely say, "It's just a scratch!" We all have wellness blind spots. That's what makes it so hard to answer the question, "How are you doing? Honestly? How are you, spiritually, relationally, emotionally, vocationally?" In the next few chapters, we'll examine not only why no one is as self-aware as they need to be, but also why church workers are especially prone to cracks in our pots that leak God's precious gift of joy, our fuel for ministry.

WHAT'S DIFFERENT ABOUT CHURCH WORKERS?

Many parish professionals and Christian educators have difficulty acknowledging the depth of their own brokenness. We get pretty good at assessing the members of the flock in classroom and church, but we get equally skilled at hiding our own places of pain. We think, wrongly, that part of the job description is to present a carefully edited version of ourselves, because, after all, "I work for Jesus, for heaven's sake!" The challenge is to recognize when, like Elijah, our brokenness has knocked us off balance and then to find ways to stop tumbling toward the broom tree, to assess our degree of wellness/brokenness and to seek the healing touch of grace that we need to be restored to a greater level of health. Some churches do a great job of attending to the wellbeing of their called workers, but they are a small minority

There's an African proverb that says, "When the chief is sick, the whole village is sick!"[24] The called workers in a church are Satan's first target for spiritual assault. Ministry suffers and the whole church is hurt when its called servants are suffering.

I get it that congregations aren't sensitive to the link between worker wellness and congregational health, but I don't get it that so many of our workers don't see the connection. A church's ministry team needs to be the first to recognize that everyone in the church is served better by those who enter their daily tasks spiritually strong, whispering the prayer, "Thank you, Lord, for rest, for strength, for the joy of this opportunity, for a receptive congregation, and for time alone with you to prepare for this great work!"

There are serious threats to spiritual, relational and vocational wellness that are unique to church workers. We're going to take a close look at some

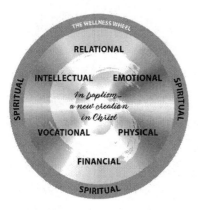

of them in these next three chapters using The Wellness Wheel as our guide. At Grace Place Wellness Ministries, in our work of nurturing wellness in the midst of the curse of brokenness, we use The Wellness Wheel[25] as a model, a paradigm for self-awareness that outlines eight important aspects of a healthy, balanced life. The eight[26] aspects of wellness depicted in the model serve as an outline for much of

this book, as they do for our retreat programming. For the sake of simplicity and clarity, we've clustered the various aspects of church worker wellness into three groups that share a commonality. Those three clusters form the subjects of this chapter and the two that follow. Baptismal and Spiritual Wellness (the hub and the rim of The Wheel) will be considered together in this chapter under the heading "Life with God." Relational, Intellectual and Emotional Wellness will similarly be treated as a group in the next chapter, "Life in Community." Finally, Vocational, Physical and Financial Wellbeing will be brought together in the subsequent chapter under the heading of "Life in Ministry."

The next three chapters come with a warning: this can get a bit discouraging. We're going to examine why the joy of life with God, the joy of life in community and the joy of life in ministry can be so easily depleted from the lives of church workers, and often, their families.

Health care workers in training study a new list of diseases each day, then meet after class and discuss, "I think I have that!" Please don't panic when studying these next three lessons. You don't have every malady we'll discuss. Our experience with thousands of church workers is that most all of us can identify one significant issue that most hinders our wellness. We encourage everyone to approach these chapters with the intention of discovering that one primary place where they are feeling depleted and focus on that aspect of life to find the Lord's healing, sustaining grace.

> We encourage everyone to seek to discover that one primary place where they are feeling depleted

And please remember: this is a survey of the broad and expansive variety of forces at work that hinder church worker wellness. Your task is to find that one golden nugget, that one "Aha!" moment that helps you identify the most critical place in your life where you need the Lord's healing touch. If you're ready, please proceed on your adventure to joy in ministry!

Let's examine some of the forces at work that have the potential to crack these frail pots of ours, forces that illustrate Lesson Six: Ministry threatens the joy of life with God.

LIFE WITH GOD

Moses hid in a cleft in the rock when the presence of the Lord passed by because standing in the holy and awesome glory of God would have meant certain doom, but the presence of God in our lives doesn't mean doom for us. By grace, we stand boldly in the presence of the glory of God every moment of our existence. "In [Christ] and through faith in him we may approach God with freedom and confidence" (Ephesians 3:12).

It's a beautiful gift to live and move and journey through life wrapped in the wonder and comfort of God's perfect, immeasurable love, and not just to live there, but to have the calling to proclaim that his love is for everyone. It's a wonderful gift, but even church workers have those moments and those days when we forget that no matter what we're enduring, God is faithful, loving us all the way through, just as he loved and carried Elijah through his trial to a new beginning. There are a thousand forces at work in our lives every day that would cause us to forget God's faithfulness. We're all subject to those moments of doubt. Your call to service in the church does not impart immunity. It seems odd, but the reality of ministry life is that those who remind others of the love of God also need to be reminded every day. The problem is ironic because in the midst of sharing the hope of Christ with others, we can fall into the trap of neglecting the faith sustaining Word in our own lives. A temptation for every follower of Christ, the problem is compounded by forces that are unique to church workers: the nature of the demands of this ministry lifestyle. It's why ministry threatens the joy of life with God.

BAPTISMAL BROKENNESS

Baptismal brokenness is when we forget who we are: a new creation in Christ. Sometimes it seems that the whole world is conspiring to make church workers lose their identity, similar to the way that Satan tempted Jesus in the wilderness (see Matthew 4:1-11; Luke 4:1-13). Think of all the messages we receive in the course of a week telling us that "You're different. You're not like all the rest!" almost as if the devil were taking us into the wilderness and whispering in our ear, "If you are truly a minister of the gospel…" Every one of those messages includes a subtle temptation to dress up in the glittering image, the old sinful nature gilded in the appearance of "having it all together." Every one of them is intended to make us forget our baptismal identity and assume an identity that is far more fragile and vulnerable to assault. Have you ever noticed the subtle little temptation in these messages, designed to define yourself differently than others?

- ▶ You're expected to dress just a bit more conservatively than others, and expected to avoid "objectionable" material in your viewing habits. You're different.

- ▶ Church leaders at budget time are heard to say, "They don't care about the money. That's why they work at a church!" You're different.

- ▶ Young people in your classroom seem shocked to discover that you have passions, interests and opinions, and that you "have a life" outside of school. You're different.

- ▶ Friends from "back home" see you and ask, "Don't you teach religion or something?" You're different.

- ▶ You're told to "be careful" on social media because "people are watching." You're different.

- ▶ People laughing at an off color joke change the subject when you approach. You're different.

Church workers find themselves in an unusual identity conundrum: their personal identities, who they are as they stand before God, and their professional identity, who they are as they stand before people, are intimately intertwined with their baptismal identity. It can become difficult to reconcile who we are as called, commissioned professionals in ministry and who we are as children of God under the cross. Do I speak words of blessing and encouragement because I'm your friend in Christ and I love you, or because "That's what you're supposed to do"? Am I acutely conscious of my intake of alcohol at a social gathering because it's part of my Christian discipline, or is it because the crowd is acutely aware of how much "The Religious Person" is drinking? Do I expect my children to be in Sunday School each week because it's part of their spiritual nurture or because I know how I'll feel if someone notices them missing? How often do we struggle with these questions because our motivation is some muddled combination of both our identity in Christ and our calling into ministry?

Sometimes these quandaries hit us openly and blatantly enough that we can recognize them and confront them. "Hey, that's not fair! It's me in here, and I'm nothing but a redeemed sinner like you, no different than anyone else!" At other times this confused identity rumbles around inside at a much deeper, unidentified level where it slowly gnaws away at our baptismal wellbeing. At our worst, we wake up one morning unable to separate our Christian walk with God from the duties and responsibilities of our work in the Church. Professional church workers can easily slip into the common error of confusing their baptismal identity in Christ with their occupational/vocational identity as ministers of the gospel. It's easy to begin to identify our worth in God's eyes with what we do for him, rather than by what he's done for us.

Baptism is God's power at work transforming our identities. It's "the washing of rebirth and renewal by the Holy Spirit" (Titus 3:5) who has made us "a new creation; the old has gone, the new has come" (2 Corinthians 5:17). By baptism into Christ, we are delivered from who we used to be, lost, condemned creatures under the wrath of God, and made into someone new; forgiven children welcomed into the family of God, loved, cherished and redeemed by His saving grace. Our new creation identity as children of God

> "Do not rejoice that the spirits submit to you, but rejoice that your names are written in heaven" (Luke 10:20)

is constantly under assault. For church workers, the temptation to find our identity in what we do for God, the functions of ministry, is an occupational hazard and a direct attack on our baptismal identity. It's why ministry threatens the joy of life with God. Jesus warned the disciples, "Do not rejoice that the spirits submit to you, but rejoice that your names are written in heaven" (Luke 10:20).

This truth bears repeating: If I find my identity in what I do for God, rather than in what he has done for me, the work of the gospel in my life is threatened, my faith is threatened, my security that rests only in his grace is threatened, the joy of walking in faith with God is threatened and I'm in danger of a collapse under the broom tree. People in the ministry professions owe it to one another to gather together around the Word of God, to have open and honest conversations about how law and gospel apply to us, and to help each other safeguard our identities as redeemed and forgiven sinners under the cross. We don't try this alone!

How well does (or doesn't) this section describe your current circumstance?

| *"Thank you, Lord. That's not my current wellness challenge."* | 1 | 2 | 3 | 4 | 5 | 6 | *"Lord, have mercy. That describes precisely what I'm enduring."* |

Note to self:

Vigilance over our baptismal identity in Christ is central to survival in ministry and our spiritual wellbeing. It requires daily renewal and restoration. Restoring our frail and damaged identities as children of God is a moment by moment happening through the course of the day, a "right now" kind of event.

It's deeply grounded, however, in the life-long "every day of my life" journey of spiritual nurture in Word and Sacrament, the closely related second aspect of our life with God.

SPIRITUAL BROKENNESS

If baptismal wellbeing is a moment by moment dying and rising to be refreshed in my identity as God's beloved, spiritual wellness is the ongoing, daily and lifelong feeding and refreshment of the soul through the means of grace. Spiritual brokenness is a result of deprivation; a starvation diet of God's Word.

Just like every other child of Adam who walks the earth, church workers are born spiritually impoverished, absolutely devoid of the nourishment that only God the Holy Spirit can provide and which he has chosen to provide for us through his Word. When lives are transformed, God gets all the credit. He is the Potter; we are the clay. We call this a "receptive theology."[27] Our lives, our spirits, are like unfashioned vessels and we are incapable of finding or providing for the nurture of our souls without the exclusive work of God himself, the only provider of faith, truth, wisdom and every other good spiritual gift from above. Our role in this spiritual receptivity is purely in response to the God-given gift of faith that enables us to see how desperately hungry and thirsty we are for the good things of God. We respond to the call of God by simply recognizing our spiritual emptiness and answering his invitation to feast and to drink deeply of the nurture he works in Word and Sacrament. We come hungry and empty, receptive to his provision. We humbly and thankfully welcome God's work in our lives; strengthening faith, correcting error, and instilling wisdom.

Imagine for a moment a scene from your own kitchen, right next to the sink and the water faucet. Imagine a row of cups, lined up along the counter, each of them empty, but waiting to be filled. Now imagine a water pitcher, gently and generously tending to each of the empty cups, one by one, pouring out the life giving water from the faucet until each and every cup is filled.

Notice that as each cup is filled, something is happening to the pitcher. It's experiencing the joy of being a vessel in the Master's hand, gladly and freely offering itself in service so that the empty cups might be filled, but something else is happening simultaneously: the pitcher itself is becoming depleted.

Look again at the cups, pitcher, and faucet. Which one is the most critically important? Of course, it's the faucet! Unless the pitcher is returning over and over again to the steady stream of water flowing from the fountain, the work of passing on the life-giving water comes to a halt. Ministry is great, but hard. It's a constant pouring out so others might be filled, and sometimes it threatens the joy of life with God, the life of constant refreshment by his grace.

While many church workers have rich and vibrant spiritual lives of devotional reflection and worship, many others are not as diligent about welcoming and receiving the life-giving nourishment of the means of grace. In our experience at Grace Place Wellness, what we know about the spiritual lives of pastors applies equally to all categories of professional church workers. The Barna report on The State of Pastors reports from their extensive research that "[W]hile only one in 20 is at high risk of spiritual difficulties (5%) – giving the impression that this is a non-issue for most pastors – an unexpected six in 10 fall into the medium risk category (61%), suggesting there are currents worthy of notice just below the placid spiritual surface."[28] These pastors at significant risk indicated that one or more of the following correctly identified their spiritual condition:

- ▸ My spiritual wellbeing is average, below average or poor.

- ▸ It is somewhat or very difficult to invest in my own spiritual development.

- ▸ I receive spiritual support from peers or a mentor only several times per year or less.

- ▸ My tenure at my current church has not deepened my own relationship with Christ.[29]

We expect the same is true for most other church workers.

Failure to remain open and receptive to the personal nurturing of the Word of God can be a professional hazard for church workers for some of the same reasons that our baptismal identity is often placed in jeopardy. Hunger for the Word of God comes from a place of deep humility and desperate need. It comes from the humble awareness that the price paid for pouring out my time and energy filling the empty cups of those I serve with the gospel of Christ's love is an emptiness of my own, a depletion of the pitcher that needs constant attention and refilling at the fount of God's Word. Luther warned church workers, "Let me tell you this. Even though you know the Word perfectly and have already mastered everything, you are daily under the dominion of the devil, and he does not rest day or night in seeking to take you unawares and to kindle in your heart unbelief and wicked thoughts against these three and all the other commands. Therefore you must constantly keep God's Word in your heart, on your lips, and in your ears."[30]

So how could someone in a church work profession ever lose their daily hunger for personal nurture in the Word? Sometimes it's a simple matter of complacency, a particularly dangerous occupational hazard for church workers. Since we spend so much of our time in a church, surrounded by Christian people, talking about matters of the faith, preparing for or teaching the Word of the Lord, praying for the needs of people, there's a temptation to think that our needs for personal devotional time, worship and prayer are taken care of. Some teachers tell us that they engaged in more deeply intimate conversations about the faith with co-workers at public schools than they ever did at the Christian schools they served!

It's not uncommon for people in ministry to develop an over-inflated measure of their own spiritual maturity. We can easily equate theological education with spiritual maturity. Failure to recognize the difference between "information," that is, a solid grasp on the doctrines of the church, and "formation," the Holy Spirit's healing and strengthening work on the soul, can lead to spiritual malnutrition.

Church workers run the risk of professionalizing their study of the Bible. I keep a small booklet near my desk called, "Children's Letters to God." One little fellow insightfully queried in his letter to the Lord, "Dear God, Is Reverend Coe a friend of yours, or do you just know him through business?"[31] Ouch. If communicating the truths of God's Word to students in the classroom or participants in the Bible class becomes our primary reason for opening and studying the scriptures, that is, for

> "Dear God, Is Reverend Coe a friend of yours, or do you just know him through business?"

"business," then the Word of God, which does its work by penetrating to the deepest places of the heart, skips the heart of the teacher and jumps right to the lesson plan. If the only time a teacher of the faith is engaged with the Word of God is preparation for classroom or Bible class responsibilities, the joy of life with God is threatened.

The question often asked by church workers is whether or not Bible study in preparation for ministry responsibilities is also personal spiritual formation. Personally, I think that it can be, and it should be, but it will not necessarily be so if one's personal devotional life of receptivity to the Word outside of church or classroom responsibilities is not firmly established in the quiet hours alone with God and his Word of law and gospel. The foundation of a strong personal devotional life will enhance the likelihood that time in the Word for professional responsibilities will also be as personally enriching as it can be. Time in the Word together with the other members of the ministry team, and as a member of a small group, are also important safeguards of spiritual wellbeing.

Reclaiming the Joy of a Church Vocation

Before teaching God's Word to others, it's always a good idea to ask yourself, "Has this Word from the Lord made a difference in my life this week?" Notice that it's both a question of baptismal identity and spiritual maturity. Before proclaiming law and gospel to those who gather thirsty for the Word, all teachers of the Word must first drink deeply because they know that they are just as thirsty. Professional church workers are just as guilty of unrepented sin, just as desperately in need of a word of grace as everyone else who meets at the foot of the cross; just as unworthy, and then, by the power of the gospel, just as redeemed and refreshed as all who have gone before us and all who assemble for study, worship and prayer. The temptation to think that we're somehow different because we bear the titles and trappings of ministry, that we are somehow exempt from the condemnation of the law or the healing power of the gospel is what puts our life with God in jeopardy. It has the potential to rob us of our heritage of joy and to land us under the broom tree. That's precisely the warning of Lesson Six: ministry itself threatens the joy of life with God.

A church worker taking time away to tend to his own spiritual wellbeing described it this way: "I feel so distant from God. One of the greatest mistakes of [ministry] is to think that because you work for God, you're close to God."[32]

Just as Elijah was caught off guard by the forces at work threatening his life with God, many church workers have a hard time admitting that their own spiritual life is susceptible to decay. Most members of the congregation would be shocked and surprised, maybe horrified, to know the struggles that so many called church workers experience in their own spiritual lives. They shouldn't be. Your personal spiritual health is a frontline battleground between the forces of evil and the Spirit of the living God. Your baptismal and spiritual health is fragile and under constant assault, but it's critical to the life, health and mission of the church. Satan attacks the church at the place where it's most vulnerable. The only defense is a rich, Christ-centered, Spirit-led life of Word and Sacrament.

How well does (or doesn't) this section describe your current circumstance?

"Thank you, Lord. That's not my current wellness challenge."   **1   2   3   4   5   6**   *"Lord, have mercy. That describes precisely what I'm enduring."*

Note to self:

A WORD OF HOPE

The good news is that there is Someone who knows us perfectly, better than we know ourselves, who is never confused about where we stand with him and why we stand boldly in his presence. The same Lord who remained faithful while Elijah drifted into doubt and despair is faithfully by your side, too. In his Word God has given us a mirror to see ourselves with the same absolute clarity with which he sees us. The mirror of God's Word comes to us first in the law, the great equalizer that reminds us that even though we wear the mantle of the holiest office, we are no different than anyone else. And then the light of the gospel reminds us of the amazing grace of Christ and gives us the eyes of faith to see ourselves the way our Father sees us, beloved and redeemed. We might be tempted to use the cultural assessment tools of popularity, economics, influence or good looks to judge how we're doing, but we do much better by looking to the Lord and his gift of baptismal grace.

Following this chapter, we'll take a short break to consider how the Bible describes what a healthy baptismal and spiritual life for church workers looks like. Those depictions of wellness will later serve as your springboard to developing a wellness plan of your own.

In Lesson Four, "Don't try this alone!," I intentionally highlighted the congregation's role in the spiritual wellbeing of church workers. The body of Christ depends on every member living together in trust, respect and love. Church workers are at the hub of the interrelated network of dozens and sometimes hundreds of relationships in the church, and that can make it a relationally dangerous place to be. Lesson Seven will highlight the particular relational hazards of professional church workers.

NOT FINISHED YET!

Take a few minutes to consider whether Lesson Six, "Ministry threatens the joy of life with God" is a lesson about ministry that you've taken to heart.

» What did you read in this chapter that resonates most deeply? What made you say to yourself, "That's really true!"?

» How would you phrase Lesson Six differently?

» What did Darrell not discuss in this chapter that really could have been mentioned?

» If this is a lesson you've already learned from your own experience, when did you first discover that it was true?

» What needs your further contemplation before moving on to the next chapter?

MINISTRY TEAM CONVERSATION STARTERS FOR LESSON SIX

» What's it like to be a "professional Christian"? How could a career in ministry cause confusion of your baptismal and vocational identities?

» How real is this threat: "If I find my identity in what I do for God, rather than in what he has done for me... the joy of walking in faith with God is threatened"?

» Tell about a time when you were so busy doing the Lord's work that you forgot about the Lord.

» Explain the analogy of the faucet, the pitcher, and the cups. What other analogy would you use to describe Lesson Six?

» What do you do to remind one another of your baptismal identity in Christ?

» When is your ministry at its best studying God's Word together?

The Biblical Design for Life with God

BAPTISMAL WELLNESS

In One Word: IDENTITY

(The Fruit of the Spirit is LOVE)

My confidence by faith that moment by moment, in every triumph, God's LOVE (Gal. 5:22) is my abiding, comforting reality and source of joy.

A Word from Ephesians 4:21-24

Surely you heard of him and were taught in him in accordance with the truth that is in Jesus. You were taught, with regard to your former way of life, to put off your old self, which is being corrupted by its deceitful desires; *to be made new* in the attitude of your minds; and to put on the new self, created to be like God in true righteousness and holiness.

Summary Marker of Baptismal Wellness

As I grow in God's grace of Baptismal LOVE,
I am finding joy in my IDENTITY as his new creation in Christ.

The JOY of Life with God is interrupted when stress and anxieties of life in a fallen world distract me from God's outpouring of grace.

Baptismal Wellness is the healing touch of Christ restoring the joy of living in my Baptismal Identity, by the Holy Spirit's gift of Love.

Growth in the Baptismal life is learning to die to self daily, moment by moment, and to rise again, a new creation in Christ.

Baptismal Wellness in Churches happens when the local body of Christ puts off the desires of the old nature and lives together according to the new nature in Christ.

Additional Scriptures: Titus 3:4-7; Romans 6:1-11; Luke 15:11-32; Psalm 23

Biblical examples of Baptismal Wellness: Peter (John 20:15-19); Paul (Philippians 3); Prodigal Son (Luke 15:11-32)

Narrative Description of Baptismal Wellness

Have you ever had a day where nothing went right? You might have had a day like that this week! Maybe you wake up in physical pain every day, and it follows you every waking hour. Maybe a few ill-spoken words led to a spat with someone you love. It changes your day. Someone has disappointed you. Car trouble. Bad news comes; bad news of illness, or heartbreak, or loss.

Jesus told of two brothers in Luke chapter 15. One lived a prodigal life, and when everything crumbled, his father's love restored the joy of living. His brother, who had never left home, also needed renewal in his father's love as he called out, "What about me?" When our expectations for a great day unravel for any reason, we also have a Father who is waiting, loving, redeeming and restoring us.

That's Baptismal Wellbeing. Whenever the thought of handling life's challenges and disappointments begins to overwhelm us with stress and anxiety, we flee once again to the waters of Holy Baptism. There, in the midst of life's traumas, we are reminded, "You are not alone. I have redeemed you. You are my own dear child. Right in this very moment, I am loving you, blessing you. I am with you. You will not have to handle this alone."

Every Christian is invited to return to their baptism a thousand times a day, if necessary. What a difference it would make in our lives if we remembered even once or twice each day to pause, be refreshed in the promise of God's gracious presence, the promise of his love, to whisper quietly, "Lord, have mercy," and then, in the power of the Spirit, faithfully face the challenges our loving Father has allowed to come our way.

SPIRITUAL WELLNESS

In One Word: RECEPTIVITY
(The Fruit of the Spirit is GOODNESS)

I welcome the transformative work of the Holy Spirit through Word and Sacrament as he builds in me GOODNESS (Gal. 5:22), the character of Jesus Christ.

A Word from Ephesians 4:13-16

...until we all reach unity in the faith and in the knowledge of the Son of God *and become mature,* attaining to the whole measure of the fullness of Christ. Then we will no longer be infants, tossed back and forth by the waves, and blown here and there by every wind of teaching and by the cunning and craftiness of men in their deceitful scheming. Instead, speaking the truth in love, we will in all things grow up into him who is the Head, that is, Christ. From him the whole body, joined and held together by every supporting ligament, grows and builds itself up in love, as each part does its work.

Summary Marker of Spiritual Wellness

As I grow in God's grace of Spiritual GOODNESS,
I am finding joy in RECEPTIVITY to his gifts, maturing and
growing in Christ.

The JOY of Life with God is interrupted when my neglect of the Word and Sacraments and the spiritual disciplines leaves me depleted of God's means of grace.

Spiritual Wellness is the healing touch of Christ restoring the joy of living in Spiritual Receptivity, as the Holy Spirit builds the character of Christ by his gift of Goodness.

Growth in the Spiritual life is learning to welcome the work of God in me as I grow toward maturity, the whole measure of the fullness of Christ by his Word.

Spiritual Wellness in Churches happens when the local body of Christ is joined and held together, growing mature in Christ by corporate study of God's Word.

Additional Scriptures: 2 Timothy 3; 2 Corinthians 5:14-17; 2 Corinthians 3:17-18; Psalm 119

Biblical examples of Spiritual Wellness: David (2 Samuel 11-12); Saul/Paul (Acts 9); Elijah (1 Kings 19); The Berean Church (Acts 17:10-12); The Emmaus Disciples (Luke 24:13-35).

Narrative Description of Spiritual Wellness

Aaron knew what God smelled like. The high priest was allowed to enter the most holy place, the place of God's presence, scented with a special aromatic perfume that had anointed all the sacred articles, a perfume used only for the things kept in that sacred place, including the high priest, Aaron himself.

Have you ever been jealous of the twelve disciples who also knew what Jesus smelled like? Every day they watched Jesus enter a crowd or enter a room and change everything just by his presence, by the "fragrance" he brought with him. By his words and actions, everything was different when Jesus showed up.

Aaron left the presence of God and moved among the people bearing a special fragrance. That's the calling of all Christians: *"For we are to God the pleasing aroma of Christ ..."* (2 Corinthians 2:15). You probably know people who bear the fragrance of Christ, who enter a room and by their words of peace, hope, joy and encouragement, who by their acts of love and compassion, change the atmosphere. They bear Christ with them wherever they go.

The only way to be bearers of Christ's presence is to be in his presence by Word and Sacrament. Spiritual Wellness is a life that's defined not by our holiness or goodness, but by the work of God the Spirit in us through his means of grace. We become less and Jesus becomes greater when we are humbly receptive to his Word of law and gospel that transforms and matures us.

A devotional life of worship, study and prayer is central to the wellbeing both of individual Christians and Christian communities. We are and always will be people of the Word. There we find the presence, power and fragrance of Christ.

MINISTRY TEAM CONVERSATION ON THE "LIFE WITH GOD" WELLNESS ASSESSMENT

Discuss together the "Markers of Wellbeing" as they apply to your Ministry Team's corporate wellness.

Summary Marker of Baptismal Wellness

As I grow in God's grace of Baptismal LOVE,
I am finding joy in my IDENTITY as his new creation in Christ.

Summary Marker of Spiritual Wellness

As I grow in God's grace of Spiritual GOODNESS,
I am finding joy in RECEPTIVITY to his gifts,
maturing and growing in Christ.

7

And Ministry Threatens the Joy of Relationships

ELIJAH SAID, "I AM THE ONLY ONE LEFT" (1 KINGS 19:9-10). The isolation of ministry crushed him. At his lowest point, curled up in a cave on Mount Horeb, God asked, "What are you doing here, Elijah?" After recounting the history of Israel's apostasy, the reason he gave for his collapse was loneliness. They're the saddest words in this heartbreaking story of ministerial burnout: I am the only one left.

There's no indication in the 1 Kings narrative that Elijah had the comfort of close family ties; in fact, his three years in the widow's home hint at just the opposite. Had he nowhere else to go? From his point of view, his peers in ministry had likewise disappeared and the community of a faithful remnant had vanished. He felt utterly alone.

It should be no surprise to us then that God's words of restoration and renewal to Elijah focused specifically on surrounding him with a close network of relationships, both in the broader fellowship of the faithful and in a closer network of ministry partners. When the Lord dusted him off and sent him back to the harvest fields, he sent the prophet with instructions to anoint new kings and a partner in the prophetic call, Elisha; to rediscover that he was not alone in his faithfulness to God's covenant promises. There were seven thousand in Israel who had not bowed down to the Baals.

Elijah's restoration to vitality and joy in ministry was a restoration to the joy of fellowship, walking in faith and service with others.

The sad tale of isolation in ministry continues to plague church workers today. On the second page of the Bible, the Lord God said, "It is not good for the man to be alone," (Genesis 2:18) and that truth is affirmed on nearly every page that follows. The scriptures clearly teach our need for fellowship, but loneliness is a chronic affliction for many of those who teach the scriptures. Ministry is an isolating profession. It's ironic that our business is people, but the nature of the business, the uniqueness of the profession, actually works against the intimacy of close relationships. We stand at the intersection of the complex web of relationships that constitute church life, but often feel all alone.

God gave us the institutions of family and church for our benefit, to help make us as fully human as we can be. The Creator also designed us for close friendships with our peers, and when Jesus sent the disciples out two by two, a practice followed by the apostles after Christ's Ascension, he instituted team ministry for his kingdom workers. We're at our best, our healthiest, when we're in this together as families, churches and partners in ministry. Remember: "Don't try this alone!" Lesson Seven on the journey to vitality and joy in ministry states, "And ministry threatens the joy of life in community."

LIFE IN COMMUNITY

Think back on your own most joyous times in life. If you're like most of us, your greatest moments of celebration are shared with others in your family, with friends, in team victories, and in your church as you look together with one heart and one set of eyes and say, "God is in the midst of us! Look at the wonders he has performed!"

The harsh reality of life in our communities of faith, however, is that our differences can also be the greatest challenge to our unity. We confess, "one Lord, one faith, one birth"[33] with all others who join us at the foot of the cross because we're united by the same human malady: our sinful, mortal, weak human nature. We're also united by the same hope that the perfect Son of God gave himself for all of us and for every one of us. By the same faith, given by the same Spirit, the members of the body of Christ are brought together to live in communities of peace: families, friendships, congregations, and ministry teams.

And at the center of God's wild mix of diversity, you are called to be a builder of unity. Keep the faith, keep everyone happy, keep the peace. How's that working out?

Paul taught the Ephesians that the seemingly impossible has become possible through Christ. Because of the gospel of grace and forgiveness, the barriers that separate have been brought down. Even the "dividing wall of hostility" that separated Jews and Gentiles was broken down (Ephesians 2:14). Brought near to God in Christ, we are brought near to one another also.

But still, harmony with "one another" is so difficult that the New Testament talks about it almost constantly. Lesson Seven, "Ministry threatens the joy of life in community," forces us to examine the difficulty of managing healthy human relationships, our life in community with others. In this chapter we'll look at the forces at work that make harmony with others such a challenge for church workers who find themselves swimming in a sea of the anxiety that characterizes some of the most intense relationships on earth: people in congregational community.

OUR VARIOUS COMMUNITIES

Church workers learn to balance complex relationships of three or four different kinds in order to thrive in their calling: 1) our own marital and family relationships, 2) our network of close friendships, 3) our congregational relationships with those we serve and, for those who work in multiple staff ministries, 4) our ministry team partnerships.

We'll examine each of these four communities under three categories found on The Wellness Wheel: Relational, Intellectual and Emotional Wellness.

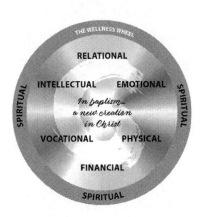

Church workers thrive when their various communities live in UNITY, (Relational Wellness); when their communities exhibit a healthy CURIOSITY about one another and when they communicate well (Intellectual Wellness); and when their communities seek to restore HARMONY when the peace is broken (Emotional Wellness). At the end of the chapter, after looking at the obstacles to Relational, Intellectual and Emotional Wellness, you'll find an overview of what the scriptures teach about God's intention for wholeness in each of those arenas.

Let's examine how each of these three, Relational, Intellectual and Emotional wellness, are threatened in each of our four relational communities because of the uniqueness of life in ministry.

MINISTRY THREATS TO RELATIONAL WELLNESS

Relational Wellness and Families

While pastors tend to be married at a rate higher than the national average, that's not necessarily so for non-ordained church workers. Most people in ministry occupations know stories of "The Fishbowl;" living under the constant scrutiny of those we serve. The public nature of what we do puts our families on display. This kind of scrutiny makes it extraordinarily difficult for single church workers to navigate the delicate waters of dating relationships with an appropriate amount of privacy. Single church workers are prime targets for anyone who has the "matchmaker" impulse. Not only are there dozens who would suggest the perfect match, there are often many more who, when a relationship becomes publicly known, are ready to offer their opinion about the suitability of the potential love interest.

Single church workers also have a tendency to serve in places some distance from their families of origin, often a considerable distance. Explaining to parents and friends that God, in his wisdom, has placed them far from home creates an extra level of anxiety that married workers may not experience as intensely. Faithfulness to the call and a desire to plant roots is complicated by the question, "Where's home?" Ministry is an isolating profession, and especially so for single church workers.

I loved the life of a parish pastor, but I sometimes hated what it did to the unity I desired in my marriage and family life. One early study of church worker burnout labelled this tension "the conflicting loyalties of church and home."[34] The tension often begins long before a couples' time of service in that first congregation and sometimes while they are still considering the call into ministry. When I asked Carol to marry me, my first year at seminary was already on the horizon, so she told me, "I don't play piano. I don't teach Sunday School. I'm not the President of the Ladies Guild and I certainly will never wear my hair in a little bun on top of my head!" I think she had a better understanding than I did of the strain on our marriage that the demands of ministry would eventually make. The sense of God's call into church work is sometimes not equally shared by marriage partners. Some couples work through the issues reasonably well. Others fail miserably and their families suffer for it.

Reclaiming the Joy of a Church Vocation

When I entered my first parish, I knew there would be sacrifices to make. I didn't realize that my family would be making so many of them. I don't remember too many times that I considered the demands upon myself unbearable, but I do remember that the closest I ever came to leaving parish ministry were those times when my family was called upon to endure life in the fishbowl, undeserved criticism, loneliness, and the many other burdens of the church worker's family. Christian counselors tell us that church work couples in counseling will often report that the demands of the school or church present the greatest burden of care and anxiety in their relationship.

Professional church workers engage in what is commonly referred to as "a high calling," and if not managed well, family life can suffer because of it. While not often explicitly stated, many church workers place their vocational vows above their vows of marriage and family life. There are times when the family is called to make sacrifices, but when managed poorly, ministry becomes a form of idolatry.

A second contributing factor to the church versus family dilemma is the nature of the work itself. In the high calling to reach the lost souls of humanity, the harvest is never ending. The tasks of ministry seem to have the voice of the Sirens, enticing the church worker to drop all else for the sake of the next task, and the next, and the next. With existing ministries fledgling, new ones waiting to be initiated, lesson plans to be written, and papers to be graded, a church worker's mind and heart are never fully at rest. We're passionate about our callings, and our families can sense that the "quivering mass of availability" that we often are has mind and heart tuned in elsewhere. They also know how hard it is for us to be forced to choose between disappointing church members who expect our presence and disappointing our own families, and without appropriate relational boundaries in place, our families sometimes tell us to "Just go!" The call of ministry threatens the joy of life in community with our families and the gift of UNITY we celebrate in our homes.

Relational Wellness in Friendship

The Barna report notes that while church workers generally feel strongly supported by those who are close to them, they are also, "more likely than the general population to feel lonely and isolated from others."[35] That's the paradox of friendship for church workers. On the one hand, they feel that those close to them are on their side and invested in their success in ministry, but on the other hand, that professional support does not translate naturally into personal friendship and care. The report goes on to say that close friendships are critically important to church worker's satisfaction in their calling. "When it comes to having true friends, there are dynamic differences between [those] who say they are satisfied with their church and vocation and those who are not, and between leaders who fall at various points along the spiritual and burnout risk metrics. The correlations between higher friendship satisfaction and lower overall risk make a compelling case for the necessity of genuine friendships."[36]

Close friendships with congregational members can be awkward for church workers. "Can I develop a close relationship with parents of my students or people I am discipling? Will they share their lives the way friends do, or will our professional relationship interfere?" It's not impossible, but it can place both church workers and those they serve in a delicate situation.

Relational Wellness in Congregations

Called workers in the church are expected to be on friendly terms with every member of the church and to be ambassadors of peace. Every time we enter a new congregation and their long-standing and intricately woven web of relationships, we walk unknowingly into the anxiety that infiltrated church life decades before we arrived. Sometimes members of the congregation never really give the new staff member a chance to develop relationships with the church family because of mistakes made by a predecessor years or even decades before their arrival. The bonds of the longtime members are sometimes so strong that church workers and their families are treated as outsiders no matter how long they serve.

The governing Boards of churches and schools make decisions that positively or negatively affect them and their families in significant ways. There is a direct correlation between ministry satisfaction and our relationship with decision makers. There's often an awkward tension between church workers and their ministry boards. It's easy for the unity that God intends for churches and their called servants to be severely strained.

Since the time of the prophets and the apostles, ministry has provided unmatchable gifts of joy to those who know God's people, who love God's people and who serve God's people. It's sad but true that sometimes taking the role of truth tellers among God's people makes it difficult for us to establish and maintain loving and caring relationships with the members of the flock, making us feel like outsiders in the very congregation they have dedicated ourselves to serving. Lesson Seven teaches truth: sometimes ministry itself threatens the joy of life in community.

Relational Wellness in Team Ministry

When Moses followed Jethro's advice and multiplied the ministry by appointing leaders of ten, fifty, one hundred and one thousand, the conflicts that divided them were healed and the whole nation was better served (see Exodus 18), but sometimes Moses could not even work with his own sister and brother (see Numbers 12). Paul had great working relationships with Barnabas and with Timothy, but clashed with Peter and refused to take Mark on a mission trip. I've served as an associate pastor at churches where the team ministry was the greatest joy and the hardest thing to leave behind and at other churches where the team relationships were the greatest roadblock to productive ministry. What is it that makes team unity so fragile?

I can think of at least six factors that work against UNITY in multiple staff ministries. First, professional church workers are asked to produce mountains of ministry results with pebbles of staff, time, money and support resources. Classroom teachers especially struggle to find a few moments during the day to spend with each other. Second, pastors are often elevated to positions of team leadership because of their success as sole pastors in smaller congregations, but have never been equipped to manage the intricacies of leading a diverse team. The same is sometimes true of school administrators who excelled in the classroom, but prove to be poor providers of the needs of faculty and staff. Third, ministry teams are sometimes unwilling to have the stormy and awkward conversations to resolve differences that arise about mission and ministry priorities in order to find unanimity as they move forward with assigned tasks. Without the hard work of establishing the norms for teamwork, ministry gets stuck and team members grow increasingly frustrated. Fourth, individual members of ministry teams are made different. Staff members bring together a wide variety of personality types, work styles, past experiences, skill sets, training and biases from their generational background that make cohesion for the sake of the ministry very challenging. Fifth, it's very natural for professional church workers in team ministry at church and school to develop close friendships with other members of their team. It can be challenging to manage the task dynamics of "getting the job done" and still remain close with good friends on the team, all the while avoiding the pitfalls of cliques within the ministry team.

And sixth, Satan's strategy is to destroy UNITY by attacking church leaders, and the tiniest foothold of misunderstanding or disagreement among ministry team members is all the base of operations that the enemy needs to divide and conquer ministry teams. The warning of Lesson Seven, that the nature of ministry in the body of Christ threatens the joy of life together in service, is a call to constant prayer and attention to team ministry working relationships. It's also a call to strengthen lines of communication among co-workers in the church.

How well does (or doesn't) this section describe your current circumstance?

"Thank you, Lord. That's not my current wellness challenge."   1   2   3   4   5   6   *"Lord, have mercy. That describes precisely what I'm enduring."*

Note to self:

MINISTRY THREATS TO INTELLECTUAL WELLNESS

Intellectual Wellness in Families

Church workers and their families are particularly prone to breakdowns in communication. The hectic lifestyle can leave little room for the CURIOSITY that leads to the intimate conversations that keep marriage and family life fresh. Once a marriage partner or children feel neglected by time demands, resentment builds, which leads to cynicism and sarcasm in the all too infrequent daily interactions and the challenge of staying intimate is compounded. Resentment is extremely common in church work spouses and children. UNITY in family life is sustained by a constant CURIOSITY about what's happening in the lives of those we love. That's Intellectual health.

Professional concerns for confidentiality can also put a damper on communication with our spouses. It's a strain on our marriages when we know more than we can share about families in the church who are also our friends. Our silence is often received with at least some level of misunderstanding. Ministry threatens the joy of relationships when our vows of confidentiality influence our conversations at home in ways most married couples never experience.

Intellectual Wellness in Friendship

We all have a God-given need to have close friendships where we know the hurts, fears, dreams and joys of others, and are intimately known by those who care about us most. These kinds of Christian friendships are important for all church workers, whether single or married, but people in ministry are notorious for their lack of close friendships.

Intellectual Wellness, a healthy CURIOSITY about others, is at the heart of the challenge many church workers have in developing close connections. The caution that constantly restrains church workers from speaking with full disclosure hinders the growth of intimacy and compassion that is the foundation of friendships. The following questions, legitimate as they are, make it a challenge to share our true feelings and true selves with others.

▶ Should I say what I actually feel?

▶ Will my true feelings, if expressed, come back around through the church/school grapevine and haunt me?

▶ Is this person seeking true friendship, or are there ulterior motives connected to my position?

Most people who gather with friends for a day of fishing or golf are not hindered by such thoughts, but church workers are. It doesn't take too many bad experiences along these lines to produce a deep sense of caution about open disclosure and personal communication in social settings. Likewise others around us might be wondering about the difference between sharing their fears and faults with us as a friend and sharing them with a member of the church's ministry team. It can be awkward to say the least. I have a pie chart hanging on my wall that reads, "What people do when they find out I'm a Pastor during normal conversation." The chart indicates, "Oh, wow, I go to First Church. You know it?" at 5%; "Silently get awkward" 5%; "Continue normally" 5%; and "Stop cussing" 85%. It makes me wonder what else people are afraid to utter within earshot of a church worker. Like Lesson Seven has been telling us, ministry threatens the joy of open, honest communication as part of life in community with others.

Intellectual Wellness in Congregations

Because churches are breeding grounds for hurt feelings due to poor communication, the joy of life in community for church workers is always under threat.

There is great wisdom in the body of Christ. One occupational hazard for church workers is to lose their CURIOSITY about church members because of the faulty belief that they have the corner on the wisdom market. Healthy congregations are open forums where every member of the body feels free to share their ideas with the expectation that they will be heard and responded to with kindness, even if they are of a minority opinion, misinformed, uninformed or just plain wrong. When the word gets around that a church staff or faculty member is not a good listener, unwilling to hear opinions about matters of church or school life that are counter to their own, communication suffers and conflict begins to rise.

With the caution to be a good listener in mind, a church worker also needs to remember how important it is to be a good communicator, sharing their own thoughts and feelings, even in matters of opinion, with honesty and clarity. The congregation may or may not agree, but it's a danger of church life for workers to stuff and stifle their own emotions, which leads to resentment and frustration and strained relationships with the congregation.

Intellectual Wellness in Team Ministry

It's rare to hear from ministry teams that their communication is always clear and complete. I'm sure there are more, but I can think of four reasons why CURIOSITY about our co-workers that keeps UNITY alive gradually diminishes. First, we have different communication styles. Some of us appreciate well thought out, bottom line, short summary statements of what we're working on, what we need, and our progress to date. Others of us value time together to think out loud, to dream, and to explore every possible option together before making a decision. We drive each other a little bit crazy if we don't appreciate the difference of our preferred communication styles and remain curious about one another's thoughts, ideas, hopes, dreams and fears in order to ensure healthy cooperation and corporate decision making. Second, the ever moving weekly, monthly and seasonal calendar leaves us with a constant urgency to produce results; time for quality communication gets sacrificed. This is particularly challenging for school faculties where good communication among teachers and departments is so essential, but the team is so often scattered across their wide areas of responsibility that communication breaks down. Third, while the age range of team members can be a great asset, we can easily talk past each other because of our different assumptions about the world and the nature of ministry or even because of our different levels of comfort with communication technologies. And fourth, people in ministry, especially in team ministry, often fall into the temptation of protecting the glittering image of ministry successfulness which makes us unwilling to reveal our true vulnerability or to ask for help when we need it. It's Lesson Seven: Ministry that demands close relationships with others threatens the interdependence at the heart of the joy of life in ministry together.

How well does (or doesn't) this section describe your current circumstance?

"Thank you, Lord. That's not my current wellness challenge."   1   2   3   4   5   6   "Lord, have mercy. That describes precisely what I'm enduring."

Note to self:

MINISTRY THREATS TO EMOTIONAL WELLNESS

Emotional Wellness in Families

UNITY is God's gift to those he joins together as one. When we hurt one another's feelings through the little disappointments, misspoken words and unmet expectations, the atmosphere of love and kindness deteriorates into the bad mood of bitterness and resentment. Living and striving together in HARMONY, every part of the family working together, is an indicator that UNITY has been restored by forgiveness. That's Emotional health.

Of all the things that can contribute to a bad atmosphere in our homes, there's one culprit that stands out above the rest. Church workers and their families are always on display. Single church workers may struggle to find safe places to share the hurts and the discomfort unique to their situation. Unrelenting scrutiny and undeserved criticism of our words and actions can subject us and our families to a unique occupational hazard of the ministry.

Life in the fishbowl threatens the joy of family life.

Life in the fishbowl threatens the joy of family life when our godly yearning to "live a life worthy of the gospel" (Ephesians 4:1) morphs into a compulsion to present ourselves as completely proper in every word and action, perfectly obedient to every moral and ethical standard that befits the profession with never a thought, deed or slip of the tongue that would indicate that we and our families are just as human as anyone else. The name for it is "pietism," and when it rears its ugly head, it always drives a wedge between us and our families. It makes our spouses wonder, "What happened to the person that I married?"

There's a constant temptation among church workers to look past the gospel of grace and make either implicit or explicit demands on ourselves, our spouses and our children to live up to standards of behavior that are far beyond the capacity of disciples of Jesus. Piety is a healthy response to the gospel and an honest representation of the maturing Christian walk of faith. Pietism, on the other hand, is a sham of phoniness that our spouses and children should never have to tolerate. It creates a crisis of personal esteem, a feeling of constant frustration and resentment with oneself for the failure to live up to the internal demand for perfection. Pietism has a tendency to spill out of our hearts and slop all over those dear to us. When it does, the emotional mood of the home shifts, relationships are strained, and the tenderness of a loving family is no longer freely and joyful shared.

Church workers and their families are put on public display, often unfairly. Any compulsion to present a perfectly edited version of ourselves in public or in private can undercut the real intimacy and honesty that are so essential to loving, grace-filled marriages and family life. It can be a strong force that threatens the joy of life in our families.

Emotional Wellness in Congregations

Churches, just like families, have an emotional atmosphere; sometimes it's positive and uplifting, and sometimes it's negative and discouraging. The mood of a church is a reflection of the state of the relationships among the members; a bad atmosphere in the church is often a reflection of the state of the relationship between the members of the church and their called servants. Two aspects of congregational life put church workers at risk for a greater level of emotional distress than most other occupations: the way congregations make decisions and the unrealistic expectations church workers and congregations have of each other, which we'll pick up in the next chapter.

For now, let's look at decision making. Church workers and the members of the congregations they serve are often equally passionate about the ministry of the church. Such passion, when disagreements about decisions for the future of the ministry arise, becomes fuel for the friction between church and school staff and the people they serve and can quickly burst into flame, taking the HARMONY of cooperative ministry with it. It's a perfect storm for disappointment, hurt feelings, resentment and conflict. As church members and called workers strive together as one body under the blessing of the Holy Spirit, joy is the fuel that keeps the ministry engine running, but decision making far too often leads to friction which, as Lesson Seven says, threatens the joy of HARMONY in the church.

The mission of sharing Christ within the church and beyond its walls requires constant evaluation, creativity and decision making. Conversations that are not conducted in a spirit of unity and love (see Intellectual Wellness above) can lead to hurt feelings, resentment and bitterness. In the midst of the decision making process, the mood changes. Congregational anxiety over potential conflict often leads to two different kinds of bad decisions. Some decisions are made too quickly as a knee-jerk reaction to a key leader's emotional outburst. Afterwards, the meeting continues in the parking lot because the real issues were not fully resolved through conversation, debate and prayer. Some decisions are made far too slowly for fear of setting off an emotional firestorm. Delayed decisions can be just as frustrating as decisions made too hurriedly. When decisions are informed by emotions, not hijacked by them, HARMONY prevails.

Emotional Wellness in Team Ministry

Psalm 55 contains these agonizing words: "If an enemy were insulting me, I could endure it; if a foe were raising himself against me, I could hide from him. But it is you, a friend like myself, my companion, my close friend, with whom I once enjoyed sweet fellowship as we walked with the throng at the house of God" (Psalm 55:12-14).

I learned Lesson Seven, that the demands of ministry threaten the joy of serving in a team, in my first congregation. The seminary placement committee asked me, "How would you deal with a very stressful team ministry situation?" which should have been a warning that I'd been designated for a call to a congregation with a long history of staff conflict! My five years there proved to be a great learning experience (see Lesson Three: Ministry is the Way of the Cross). The senior pastor and I rarely worked in HARMONY. The strained relationship with the senior pastor and the bad atmosphere that often prevailed was a never-ending motivation for personal prayer and reflection, all the way to the time of his retirement and my departure to another ministry in a different state. I was surprised years later, upon returning to the area to serve a different congregation, to strike up a very cordial and positive, respectful relationship with my former ministry partner. When I look back on it now, I can see that after his departure from the anxieties of ministry (and my growth in maturity), we were different people and got along great.

I'm convinced that it was the demands of the ministry that we faced together that put such a strain on our earlier relationship, and when we found ourselves outside of the anxieties of church life, we became good friends. At the time of his departure into glory, his wife called and told me that one of his last requests was that I speak at his funeral service!

How well does (or doesn't) this section describe your current circumstance?

"Thank you, Lord. That's not my current wellness challenge."   1   2   3   4   5   6   "Lord, have mercy. That describes precisely what I'm enduring."

Note to self:

Lesson Seven, "Ministry threatens the joy of life in community," is an important lesson to learn as we journey toward vitality and joy in ministry. Satan's strategy begins with division, and our own sinful natures are co-conspirators, but the gospel of Christ teaches that the dividing wall of hostility has already been torn down and the gift of God to all of us, to our families, to our friendships, to our churches and to our co-workers in ministry, is the unity of the faith that unites us now and endures for all of eternity. By the power of Christ's creative, binding Holy Spirit, we have every resource to be healed of the wounds we inflict on each other. No matter how badly the strain of ministry divides, the gospel has power to heal.

The gospel of God's love and forgiveness is the healing cure for the emotional distress that plagues our homes and our families. When our Life with God is rich and deep, then Life in Community will be marked by forgiveness, actively sought and given freely in all of our relationships. When God and his grace seem distant, and when the bonds of church, family and friendship are strained, our Life in Ministry is affected.

In a last twist of irony, we turn to one more way that the joy of ministry is threatened: a life in ministry itself.

NOT FINISHED YET!

Take a few minutes to consider whether Lesson Seven, "Ministry threatens the joy of life in community" is a lesson about ministry that you've taken to heart.

» What did you read in this chapter that resonates most deeply? What made you say to yourself, "That's really true!"?

» How would you phrase Lesson Seven differently?

» What did Darrell not discuss in this chapter that really could have been mentioned?

» If this is a lesson you've already learned from your own experience, when did you first discover that it was true?

» What needs your further contemplation before moving on to the next chapter?

MINISTRY TEAM CONVERSATION STARTERS FOR LESSON SEVEN

» In what ways have you found ministry to be "an isolating profession"? How has it impacted family relationships? Relationships with church members? Ministry team relationships?

» Ministry team communication is always a challenge. What works well for your team? What tells you that your team could do better? What do you do to stay connected to one another?

» "Conflict is inevitable; enemies are optional" (Frederick Buechner). What can ministry teams do to remain friends even in times of disagreement?

The Biblical Design for Life in Community

RELATIONAL WELLNESS

In One Word: UNITY

(The Fruit of the Spirit is PATIENCE)

Enjoying the bond of trust, respect and love experienced by the body of Christ in friendship, marriage, family and church when PATIENCE (Gal. 5:22) with one another overcomes differences.

A Word from Ephesians 4:2-6

Be completely humble and gentle; be patient, bearing with one another in love. Make every effort to keep *the unity of the Spirit* through the bond of peace. There is one body and one Spirit—just as you were called to one hope when you were called—one Lord, one faith, one baptism; one God and Father of all, who is over all and through all and in all.

Summary Marker of Relational Wellness

As I grow in God's grace of Relational PATIENCE,
I am finding joy in my UNITY in Christ with spouse, family and church.

The JOY of Life in Community is interrupted when sin and selfishness, the works of my old nature, hinder and block the flow of God's love one to another.

Relational Wellness is the healing touch of Christ restoring the joy of living in Relational Unity, by the Holy Spirit's gift of Patience.

Growth in the Relational life is learning to leave behind my old selfishness so that I might cleave to others in loving relationships.

Relational Wellness in Churches happens when the body of Christ becomes a fellowship of faith united in mutually shared trust, respect and love.

Additional Scriptures: Philippians 2:1-4; 1 John 4; John 13; John 17; Acts 4; 1 Corinthians 12; Psalm 133

Biblical examples of Relational Wellness: David and Jonathan (1 Samuel 20); Naomi and Ruth (Ruth 1); The Philippian Church (Philippians 1); The Church in Acts (Acts 2, 4); Christian Marriage (Ephesians 5).

Narrative Description of Relational Wellness

In their early years, Joseph and his brothers had some issues. Competition and favoritism fractured their family into a "me vs. you" mentality. Jacob's greatest desire was for family unity. The thought of his sons scattered across the world was horrifying to him. God's design for church and family and marriage is oneness of heart and mind. The gospel of Christ transforms us from a collection of "MEs" into one body, a "WE."

Healthy Christian marriages soon discover the power of two becoming one flesh, the power of "WE." The Son of God willingly let go of his personal rights and privileges in order to be our Suffering Servant and to fulfill his mission as

Savior of the world. His call to us includes self-sacrificing love, leaving the old sinful nature's living for "ME," for the blessing of unity in marriage, family and church; living as "WE."

The temptation to think first about self confronts us moment by moment throughout the day. At home we resent having to do the dirty, thankless tasks. We want the last cookie, the remote control and someone else to do the dishes. At church we expect to have our way on every important decision.

Relationships with a high level of mutual trust, respect and love are characterized by daily contrition and repentance so that the old sinful nature is put away and the new nature in Christ, marked by self-sacrifice and concern for the whole body, comes alive. Unity is a gift of God's Spirit, and a treasure to be cherished in every home and every congregation.

INTELLECTUAL WELLNESS

In One Word: CURIOSITY
(The Fruit of the Spirit is KINDNESS)

My desire to connect with others in an intimate way through honest, open sharing and listening that is guided by KINDNESS (Gal. 5:22) and sensitivity to their needs.

A Word from Ephesians 4:25, 29

Therefore each of you must put off falsehood and speak truthfully to his neighbor, for we are all members of one body.….. Do not let any unwholesome talk come out of your mouths, but only what is helpful for building others up according to their needs, that it may *benefit those who listen.*

Summary Marker of Intellectual Wellness

As I grow in God's grace of Intellectual KINDNESS,
I am finding joy in CURIOSITY, listening and speaking in a beneficial way.

The JOY of Life in Community is interrupted when prejudice, attribution of characteristics before I know others, and cutting off conversation by completing other's thoughts are all examples of selfish thinking that stifle curiosity and the bonds of love.

Intellectual Wellness is the healing touch of Christ restoring the joy of living in Intellectual Curiosity by the Holy Spirit's gift of Kindness.

Growth in the Intellectual life is learning to understand my own communication style and those of others so that I can be both a better listener and better at sharing my own heart and passions.

Intellectual Wellness in Churches happens when a spirit of discovery and the expectation of surprises and lifelong learning flows from a climate of curiosity when the body of Christ is open to everyone's ideas, dreams and wisdom.

Additional Scriptures: Acts 10; Acts 15; Acts 17; Proverbs 4; 1 Corinthians 3; 1 Corinthians 8; Psalm 139

Biblical examples of Intellectual Wellness: Peter and the Gentiles (Acts 10-11)

Narrative Description of Intellectual Wellness

Something about the Lord's hometown caused Nathanael to form an opinion. He had decided, for one reason or another, that nothing good was ever going to come from Nazareth. What an interesting surprise he got when he met Jesus. We formulate opinions about people and groups of people to make the world fit into our most comfortable notions of how things should be.

Those notions are often shattered by the facts. We enter the world with a natural, God-given curiosity. The attributions we make toward others like "I know what you're thinking!" stifle curiosity and greatly reduce the possibility of learning something, of discovery and surprise in our relationships with others.

Intellectual wellbeing is learning to show enough compassion and respect toward other people to recognize that if we would truly and sincerely listen first before forming judgments, we might just learn something. When we see everyone in our lives as a gift from God, even those we know best, curiosity will lead us to ask, "What are you thinking?" Coach John Wooden once said, "It's what you learn after you know it all that counts." That's Intellectual Wellbeing.

Some of us are hesitant to ever speak about passionate topics until we've processed our thoughts and are exactly sure what we want to say. We feel safer not displaying our emotions too quickly. Others of us jump right in, processing our thoughts aloud. We're more comfortable boldly laying our emotions out there while we get a good handle on what we're feeling. Appreciating the difference fosters good communication.

Communication is the lifeblood of relationships. Learning to listen well *and* learning to communicate our thoughts, feelings, fears and dreams well, keeps relationships lively and growing.

EMOTIONAL WELLNESS

In One Word: HARMONY
(The Fruit of the Spirit is PEACE)

Experiencing the refreshment and restoration of strained or broken relationships that comes through the healing power of forgiveness and results in PEACE (Gal. 5:22).

A Word from Ephesians 4:26, 30-32

"In your anger do not sin": Do not let the sun go down while you are still angry, and do not give the devil a foothold.... And do not grieve the Holy Spirit of God, with whom you were sealed for the day of redemption. Get rid of all bitterness, rage and anger, brawling and slander, along with every form of malice. Be kind and compassionate to one another, *forgiving each other,* just as in Christ God forgave you.

Summary Marker of Emotional Wellness

As I grow in God's grace of Emotional PEACE, I am finding joy in HARMONY with others by the healing power of forgiveness.

The JOY of Life in Community is interrupted when, like the Unmerciful Servant, failure to forgive the small debts I am owed blocks the flow of God's greater forgiveness of my unpayable debt.

Emotional Wellness is the healing touch of Christ restoring the joy of living in Emotional Harmony by the Holy Spirit's gift of Peace.

Growth in the Emotional life is learning to sincerely confess my sins to God and to those I have hurt, to be forgiven, and to fully forgive others.

Emotional Wellness in Churches happens when the local body of Christ lives together as a fellowship that takes all conflict to the foot of the cross of Jesus and welcomes the forgiveness and love he won for us.

Additional Scriptures: Matthew 18; Ephesians 2:11-22; 1 Peter 2:1-12.

Biblical examples of Emotional Wellness: Jacob and Esau (Genesis 33); Peter and Paul (Galatians 2); The Unmerciful Servant (Matthew 18)

Narrative Description of Emotional Wellness

A word spoken in anger can hang in the air for decades. A dirty trick can affect a relationship for a lifetime. No one really remembers why the Hatfields and McCoys started fighting. Everyone knew they couldn't stop.

The gospel of forgiveness in Christ heals relationships. Following a decades long grudge started by a dirty trick, brothers Jacob and Esau found forgiveness and a brand new harmony that lasted the rest of their lives. The devil likes to dig in to that place of hurt and resentment and set up his camp. He's made a lifestyle of widening a small crack in the bonds of love into the Grand Canyon of bitterness and resentment.

Our old "ME" nature enjoys getting back at other people. When we've been wronged, our natural tendency is to even the scales by throwing some hurt the other way. Revenge is sweet. Payback is a favorite pastime. But revenge and getting even destroy the "WE" in which God intends us to live.

Frederick Buechner said, "Conflict is inevitable; enemies are optional." There's no such thing as a family, a marriage or a Christian congregation devoid of disagreement and conflict. We're all people of passion with particular wants and needs, and when ours clash with those of others, storm clouds gather. Families and churches in conflict have a very difficult time moving forward in their callings to be servants of Christ to a lost and hurting world. Hurting people hurt people.

Thanks be to God that he has given us the gift of forgiveness so that we can chase the devil from our homes and churches by mutual confession, putting off the old sinful nature, and putting on Christ for one another as we learn to forgive as we have been forgiven.

MINISTRY TEAM CONVERSATION ON THE "LIFE IN COMMUNITY" WELLNESS ASSESSMENT

Discuss together the "Markers of Wellbeing" as they apply to your Ministry Team's corporate wellness.

Summary Marker of Relational Wellness

As I grow in God's grace of Relational PATIENCE,
I am finding joy in my UNITY in Christ with spouse, family and church.

Summary Marker of Intellectual Wellness

As I grow in God's grace of Intellectual KINDNESS,
I am finding joy in CURIOSITY, listening and speaking in a beneficial way.

Summary Marker of Emotional Wellness

As I grow in God's grace of Emotional PEACE, I am finding joy in HARMONY
with others by the healing power of forgiveness.

8

And Ministry Threatens the Joy of Ministry

HOW MANY PEOPLE DO YOU KNOW that began a career in church work with great enthusiasm, only to leave the ministry within a few short years?

We don't really know much about where Elijah came from or exactly how many years he served in ministry, but it's clear he was unprepared for how difficult the task was going to be. The burdens of Elijah's vocational ministry led to his mid-career collapse under the broom tree, a clear warning to everyone in the church work professions that without proper fortification of spirit, body, and family this work can take a devastating toll.

Lesson Six pointed out how ministry can be hard on the faith life of church workers. We learned in Lesson Seven that Elijah and his successors pay a heavy relational price for this calling. Ministry is an isolating profession. The relational and spiritual toll on church workers can be devastating, (see "I am the only one left"), but it could be that the primary cause of Elijah's distress, the greatest reason for his crash under the broom tree, was the very task of ministry that he was called to perform. Lesson Eight on the journey to wellness flows from Lessons Six and Seven: "Ministry itself threatens the joy of a life in ministry."

Rockford Peaches Manager Jimmy Dugan was wrong about one thing: baseball is a fun career, but it's not great. The thrill of a catch or a line drive will never compare with the joy of watching God the Holy Spirit bring his gifts of healing, renewal and joy into the lives of broken and hurting people. Baseball is cool and fun and can give moments of pleasure, but it's not great.

And if Jimmy Dugan thinks baseball is hard, it's only because he never spent years in the annual cycle of congregational life that church workers have. In a baseball game (it is a game, Jimmy!) nothing of ultimate importance hinges in the balance when a batter whiffs on a pitch or when a fielder fumbles the horsehide sphere on a sunny summer afternoon. The fans let out a Bronx cheer, guzzle down another cold frosty one, pop a few peanuts and then head back out to face real life again.

It's understandable that a life in church work would be hard on your relationships, and bewildering, although conceivable, that the ministry could be detrimental to your own personal life of faith, but the ultimate irony is that the nature of the calling into Christian service itself and the difficulty of facing the challenges inherent to the vocation could be the dominant force driving people out of service in the church. It's oxymoronic, like poisonous medicine, or a meal that leaves you hungry, but it's true. Who would have thought that the simple act of obediently following the call of God into a life of gospel service would immediately put you in jeopardy of walking away from it?

I've often counseled those considering church work careers to only go if they can't not go. This work is the way of the cross. Overwhelmed is a way of life for professional church workers. The last two chapters have been painful for me to write. Speaking the truth in love doesn't make it any easier to hear, and I know that what we've been exploring is distressing. I feel the same way about this chapter. It's hard to say, but it needs to be said. My heart's desire is for you and those around you to thrive in your callings and to experience the fullness of the Spirit's gift of joy that God intends, and if a full diagnosis of the dangers of ministry is required, then I'll say what needs to be said. I hope you'll read this chapter in the spirit in which it's offered: I want you to recognize the pitfalls of your position so that you can avoid them, or at least find your way through them a little easier. I'll review a number of those hazards, but I'm really hoping that my thoughts will trigger some of your own awareness of the unique burdens of your particular calling that only you yourself can identify.

VOCATIONAL WELLNESS IS HUMILITY

This work will humble you. Maybe God intended it that way. There's a common thread in the Bible stories of God's call into kingdom service. The greatest warriors in the advancement of the kingdom were typically the most humble right from the start. Think of those times when God called flesh and blood people like you and me. Moses said, "I could never be the guy, but I've got this brother..." Esther said, "Seriously? All I've ever done is win a beauty contest!" Isaiah said, "Here's the thing, I'm not really spokesman material because nothing good ever comes out of my mouth." Jeremiah said, "Do you really think it's a good idea to send a boy to do a man's job?" Peter said, "You better just leave, Jesus, before you make a big mistake."

Paul said it well. "Brothers and sisters, think of what you were when you were called. Not many of you were wise by human standards; not many were influential; not many were of noble birth. But God chose the foolish things of the world to shame the wise; God chose the weak things of the world to shame the strong. God chose the lowly things of this world and the despised things—and the things that are not—to nullify the things that are" (1 Corinthians 1:26-28). He's telling us, "The power of God is much easier for folks to recognize when they see how completely inadequate we are for the task." Maybe God knows what he's doing when he calls inadequate people like you and me. John the Baptist articulated it the best: "In order for everyone to get a good, clear look at Jesus, I need to stand way out of the way" (see John 3:30!)

In a word, Vocational Wellness means understanding our proper posture before the God who has called us to be the gloves on his hands. That posture is HUMILITY. Anyone who approaches the tasks of church work with an "I've got this!" attitude is in serious trouble. Maybe that's why service in the church (which is so great) is so hard (Lesson One). Maybe that's why God has made it the way of the cross (Lesson Two). Maybe that's why God allows overwhelmed to be a way of life for church workers (Lesson Three). It's so we don't try this work alone (Lesson Four), but only in the company of the body of Christ, humbly relying on the Lord's power and grace.

VOCATIONAL BROKENNESS

When we're at our best, we approach the tasks of school and church ministry with the kind of humility that C. S. Lewis was talking about when he said,

"Humility is not thinking less of yourself; humility is thinking of yourself less."

We tend to take ourselves too seriously

When we take ourselves too seriously, the forces at work that make the tasks of the call so challenging get the better of us. I see three of those forces at the top of my list: 1) the nature of the prophetic call to speak the truth with boldness; 2) the diminishing respect for religious professionals in our culture, and; 3) the unreasonable expectations that congregations have for their called workers. Let's take a look.

THE CALL TO PROPHETIC MINISTRY

A "prophet" is someone who is called to speak God's truth to a world that does not want to hear it. If you are a part of God's kingdom work in contemporary North America in a Christian school or a church, you are involved in prophetic ministry. What you have to say, people don't want to hear; neither the people of the culture around you, or sadly, often the people you serve inside the church.

Elijah in 1 Kings 19 is still the poster-boy for vocational brokenness in prophetic ministers. At Mount Carmel he discovered how great ministry can be. At Mount Horeb he fell crushed under the weight of how hard it can be. Persecuted, exhausted, lonely, afraid and despairing, Elijah learned that the prophet business can be dangerous.

Let's face it: nobody likes a prophet. Remember what we discussed back at the beginning of this journey: Jesus taught, "Blessed are you when people insult you, persecute you and falsely say all kinds of evil against you because of me. Rejoice and be glad, because great is your reward in heaven, for in the same way they persecuted the prophets who were before you" (Matthew 5:11-12, emphasis added). Don't forget what C. F. W. Walther warned his seminary students: ministers of the gospel, of all people on earth, are the "most despised and even hated by the world."[37] The gospel message of hope is generally preceded by prophetic bad news, the condemnation of the sins of sinful people, and it's not a message that sits well with folks. Our congregations call us to speak the truth. At our installations they insist that we take a solemn vow before God and the whole church that we will not compromise the message, but they often cringe, glare and even confront us directly when the truth of God's perfect law lands a little too close to home. It's agonizing for Christian church workers when the flock that called them to preach the whole Word of God becomes bitter and confrontational as the voice of the Lord calls them to repentance.

Reclaiming the Joy of a Church Vocation

Part of the prophetic message is a call to change. Christian educators in discipling ministries are often met by resistance from the most unexpected of places. You have certainly discovered by now that parochial school ministry and youth ministry are counter-cultural efforts. Not only do Christian educators find resistance and push-back from the students, they are often engaged in what seems like warfare with the parents for the hearts and minds of their own children! Called to proclaim the gospel of repentance, dying to self and rising to a new life in Christ, parents seem more interested in promoting the values of a "me first" culture in the lives of their children.

People in ministry are often uncertain whether or not their efforts are producing fruit in the lives of people. I know from my own experience and from my conversations with others that the greatest reward of our work is seeing changed lives. The problem is that a changed life is often hard to recognize and far too seldom expressed to Christian leaders. We know that church work professionals have a great desire to fill the roles of coach, healer and leader in the lives of those they serve, but are often conscripted into less threatening roles of babysitter, manager and administrator. There's a vocational risk for any profession whose practitioners exert themselves with such passion and see so few results. The danger can lead to faith struggles and can cause church workers to wonder, "Where is God in this?" The fuel tank of joy springs a leak.

When we're at our best, we serve with the conviction and confidence that our call is from God, that he is with us and working through us, and that every resource of the kingdom is at our disposal. When we're at our best, we serve out of the sincere HUMILITY of knowing that God has chosen us to be his instruments of peace and hope. The danger for those in prophetic positions is that they fail to recognize the presence of Christ's handiwork in the lives of people. That's the very definition of the absence of the joy that fuels ministry. The gravest danger for professional church workers is to lose confidence in the Lord's hand of blessing and to begin to rely more and more on our own strength and gifts and our own skill and experience. We start to function out of our own capacity. Spirit-given HUMILITY vanishes and frustration and discouragement sets in and the impossible task of ministry becomes overwhelming.

There's a broom tree waiting not far from every church worker's classroom or office.

DIMINISHED RESPECT FOR RELIGIOUS PROFESSIONALS

I'll offer just a few quick thoughts here because I expect you are well aware of how the place of clergy and other professional church workers in our society is much different than it was even just a generation ago. There was a time when church life in America was similar to the life of God's people in Old Testament Israel. Everything has changed for the new generation of church leaders. Our context is more like Ezekiel ministering to the children of God in the Babylonian exile, strangers in a strange land surrounded by a people and a culture that has no understanding of who we are or what we're trying to accomplish.

Two cultural trends have been building for decades. The first is that church workers are, by and large, irrelevant. The people in our communities do not, for the most part, care what we have to say and are not generally interested in what we think about Jesus. Especially in younger populations, Christianity and those who represent it are seen as intolerant, bigoted and narrow-minded. The second big shift in attitude toward church workers is that we are now reckoned to be untrustworthy. Financial and sexual abuse scandals among clergy and others who work with children have had a powerful influence on the perception of the character of all church workers. Once rated near the top of most trusted professions, surveys now indicate that people trust their attorney more than they trust pastors, with both registering low on the scale, and I expect that has influenced the reputations of all church workers.

The culture around us has a deeply ingrained aversion to hearing most anything that we have to say. To survive and thrive in such an environment it's important to take God's Word seriously and the power of the Spirit seriously, but in true HUMILTY of spirit, not to take ourselves so seriously. That comes from taking to heart the irony of Lesson Eight, "Ministry threatens the joy of ministry."

UNREASONABLE EXPECTATIONS

In our experience with thousands of pastors and church workers of all stripes across several decades, the unreasonable expectations placed upon church workers are far and away the number one cause of vocational discouragement. This is just as true, maybe more true, for Christian educators and other non-ordained workers in the church than it is for clergy. I expect that your mind is racing right now with the list of expectations that have been placed on your shoulders, sometimes in official job descriptions, and sometimes in demands on your time and energy that just creep in over time.

How a minister responds to unreasonable expectations is the central issue of Vocational Wellness.

Since what churches do best is carry traditions from one generation to the next, unrealistic expectations can accumulate and build over time. We've all had more responsibility scooped onto our plates. Few of us have experienced an intentional effort at reducing expectations to allow room for new tasks. This is an especially hazardous trap for single church workers. Whether explicitly stated or not, a presumption that, "She has plenty of time anyway" is disrespectful and entirely inappropriate, and can increase an already unmanageable load of responsibilities where they do not belong.

A realistic grasp of the enormity of the task should enhance the Spirit's gift of HUMILITY. Moses, Isaiah, Peter and John the Baptist were right: None of us are equipped for the task. Ideally, the staff member and the congregation will work diligently to manage the expectations of their called workers in an appropriate manner by setting priorities, calling additional staff, raising up partners in team ministry within the congregation and developing a gracious attitude toward the demands placed upon an imperfect human being. Far too often, however, church workers succumb to the expectations and work themselves into exhaustion by over-functioning; serving beyond their physical, spiritual and emotional capacity. Not only does over-functioning lead to frustration, discouragement and exhaustion on the part of the worker, the whole congregation also suffers as a called servant becomes more and more ineffective and inefficient, loses creativity, and, as noted previously, finds it increasingly difficult to recruit young people to follow in their footsteps to a life in church work.

How well does (or doesn't) this section describe your current circumstance?

"Thank you, Lord. That's not my current wellness challenge."   1   2   3   4   5   6   "Lord, have mercy. That describes precisely what I'm enduring."

Note to self:

The answers to the challenge of unreasonable expectations are not longer work days and skipped vacations or days off. Our own physical strength is the most easily exhaustible of all our resources for ministry. Let's take a quick look at why the life of ministry can be so physically debilitating to professional church workers.

PHYSICAL BROKENNESS

A concern for Physical Wellness motivates us to pursue the VITALITY of our bodies as we learn to make healthy choices about nutrition, exercise, rest and stress management. To be at our best in fulfilling our duties, we learn to live as stewards of the resources that God provides including these incredibly complex and yet exceedingly frail bodies of ours. We're also, for the sake of the work of the kingdom, called upon to manage "all the necessities and nourishment for this body and life,"[38] including our material wealth. These three are inseparably linked: Vocational, Physical and Financial Wellness. We tend to our health and our wealth so that we can give ourselves fully to the call to serve. Our physical strength and our financial capacity are limited resources that require careful management for the sake of our vocational calling.

The physical demands of the office are a significant risk factor for church workers. The needs of people are never satisfied, the lesson plans are never fully completed, and the backlog of reading material continues to climb. Every church worker knows what it feels like to be always on call, a "quivering mass of availability." When the phone rings we flip the "on" switch. Constantly being on duty leaves little room for the respite of sleep, relaxation and recreation that is vital to physical health. It's dangerous to ignore the physical limitations we're born with or those that come with age. Parish pastors exhibit higher rates of stress related illness than the general population.[39] Grace Place founder Dr. John Eckrich reports from his extensive practice serving the physical needs of church educators, musicians and their families that all church workers are likely prone to the same maladies. God designed life to be lived in daily cycles of work and rest, with an extra day of spiritual, emotional and physical rest built into every week. Failing to recognize the Lord's daily and weekly call to rest, and the cry for physical renewal often signaled to us by our own bodies, (like Elijah's body collapsing under the broom tree), is a classic sign of over-functioning.

Second, there seems to be a temptation for church workers to over-spiritualize their understanding of the physical human nature. Despite the clear teaching of the Apostles' Creed, where our physical human nature is affirmed in all three articles, a significant number of church workers seem to function out of a sort of contemporized neo-platonic philosophy, an attitude that the real self is the spiritual self, and that since the inner spiritual life with God is in sound condition through the grace of Christ, it doesn't really matter what happens to the external life of the body. Since the work of ministry is largely occupied with the spiritual life, it's easy to simply neglect matters of physical wellbeing, hoping that God will care for my body the way he cares for my soul purely as a miraculous working of his endless grace.

A cursory glance around the pastor's or educator's conference assembly hall will show a rate of obesity higher than the national average. Some studies indicate that obesity among male clergy in America exceeds the national rate by as much as 10%, and with the national rate approaching four out of ten, that's a frightening thought. Carrying too much weight puts an individual at a higher risk for a wide variety of debilitating and potentially deadly diseases. The Bible depicts a much different kind of daily lifestyle than is practiced by most church workers: hard physical labor six days a week and a largely plant-based diet, eating food the way that God designed it, not the way that Ronald McDonald did.

Churches in America are notoriously unhealthy places to work.

And finally, churches in America are notoriously unhealthy places to work. Fellowship gatherings are dominated by caffeine, fat and sugar. The board of fare at most church suppers would send many a dietician into a panic. Well-meaning but misguided parishioners show their appreciation to their called workers with a plate of cookies or a slice of pie in the middle of the afternoon, while in reality most of us would be better off with an apple, a brisk walk and a nap!

It's the responsibility of leaders in the church to teach the whole counsel of God, including a fully formed biblical anthropology, accenting the frailty of our bodies, as well as how we "thank and praise, serve and obey" our loving Creator and Sustainer through our wise stewardship of the body. The fallen sinful nature says, "It's my body; I can do anything I want with it." The new creation in Christ says, "Thank you, Lord, for this body and life. Take my hands and let them be consecrated, Lord, to Thee."

Ministry is hard. The responsibilities and corresponding schedules of most church workers are extremely taxing on their physical wellbeing. Those physical demands are part of what makes church work a threat to the joy of ministry. Church workers are people too, and we live under the same restrictions of the physical capacity of our bodies as everyone else. Jesus tended to his own physical needs for the sake of his service to others. The Spirit's fruit of self-control, poured out to restrain the lusts of the flesh, directs us toward healthier choices and VITALITY for ministry.

How well does (or doesn't) this section describe your current circumstance?

| "Thank you, Lord. That's not my current wellness challenge." | 1 2 3 4 5 6 | "Lord, have mercy. That describes precisely what I'm enduring." |

Note to self:

FINANCIAL BROKENNESS

In order to devote oneself fully to such an overwhelmingly difficult task, professional church workers need to be free of the distraction of financial worries. It's challenging to fully engage in the work of care and nurture of others when your own mind is wondering, "How am I going to pay the mortgage, finance college, retire someday?" Financial Wellness is the capacity of church workers, both financially and emotionally, to exhibit GENEROSITY even within the bounds of limited resources. That requires significant intentional work from both the church work family and the congregation.

On average, pastors are earning a living wage with pay comparable with those of similar education in the non-profit sector. That's not necessarily true of other church workers, parochial school teachers in particular, and there are still many church work families that are living near the edge of significant financial stress. Once again, some of the causes for this are external to the worker, determined by decisions made beyond their control, but other forces causing financial stress are internal and well within the church worker's influence.

I hope you've never heard this one: "We believe we should keep our worker's pay as low as possible to keep them humble."[40] Few church members seem willing to practice the same kind of humility, and most church workers I know would be even more humbled by a generous outpouring of the congregation's thankfulness through a wage comparable to the incomes of the members themselves. As outlandish as the humility comment seems, it's symptomatic of the financial concerns that are unique to church workers and their families. I've personally had finance committees suggest that I should offer to take a pay cut in order to balance the budget. That creates an awkward triangle between the worker, the congregation and the church worker's family.

Congregational leadership has a biblically mandated responsibility to be sure their workers are supported in every way, including financially. In our consultation work with churches, I ask the lay leaders four pointed questions. If you have influence with your church's leadership, I hope you are able to suggest these as questions worthy of their consideration.

1. Who reads the District's salary guidelines for workers each year? (I always wait for a response and ask them to share with the whole group what the guidelines are. In some instances, lay leaders were unaware such guidelines exist.)

2. Is your ten year trend taking you closer or further away from the guidelines?

3. Have you set a floor for salaries, a percentage of the guidelines below which salaries must not fall?

4. Are all workers treated equitably? (This question is to press the point that clergy and non-clergy and also church and school must be considered together and fairly.)

Congregational forces are not the only ones at work in the financial brokenness of professional church workers. We are often guilty of contributing to our own stress inducing financial situations. The enormous load of educational debt, combined with unusually low starting salaries, is a serious financial burden for young people in ministry. Only the most naïve of us would pursue a calling into a church work career expecting a life of wealth and luxury, but the expectation to receive a livable wage and benefits can no longer be automatic.

The burden of significant debt and low wages is compounded by some attitudinal deficiencies that are all too common in church workers and their spouses. While most have settled the issue of financial contentment with church work salaries, others still struggle with jealousy and resentment over the material sacrifices they make. The resentment over financial remuneration impacts the unity of the marriage bond. If the worker feels guilty and resentful over low wages and their spouse feels a guilt ridden reticence to complain, along with resentment about making sacrifices, and if their conversations about money commonly deteriorate into arguments, the couple avoids the difficult discussions that need to happen and poor financial decisions result. Failure to interrupt the downward slide of financial instability, particularly failure to get good advice from financial counselors or advisors, can lead to very serious financial problems. Our training institutions may or may not teach financial management, and students may or may not pay attention. Just like the unending demands of the work of ministry and the physical toll they can take, financial brokenness threatens the joy of life in ministry.

How well does (or doesn't) this section describe your current circumstance?

"Thank you, Lord. That's not my current wellness challenge."   1   2   3   4   5   6   "Lord, have mercy. That describes precisely what I'm enduring."

Note to self:

These last three chapters have been difficult to write, and I expect difficult for you to read, but the heavy burden of the impact of brokenness in ministry in Lessons Six, Seven and Eight have led us to the place of the great good news of God's healing grace that we explore in the next chapter, right after we summarize the biblical vision for Vocational, Physical and Financial Wellness.

NOT FINISHED YET!

Take a few minutes to consider whether Lesson Eight, "Ministry threatens the joy of life in ministry" is a lesson about ministry that you've taken to heart.

» What did you read in this chapter that resonates most deeply? What made you say to yourself, "That's really true!"?

» How would you phrase Lesson Eight differently?

» What did Darrell not discuss in this chapter that really could have been mentioned?

» If this is a lesson you've already learned from your own experience, when did you first discover that it was true?

» What needs your further contemplation before moving on to the next chapter?

MINISTRY TEAM CONVERSATION STARTERS FOR LESSON EIGHT

» Why is HUMILITY suggested as the attitude that safeguards vocational wellness? Tell why you agree or disagree. How has ministry humbled you?

» Rate the impact of these three of your vocational wellness, from high to low.

- The call to prophetic ministry.

- Diminished respect for church work professionals

- Unrealistic expectations

» How does your team offer encouragement and support to one another?

» What unhealthy habits could our team work to eliminate? What healthy habits could we begin to adopt?

» What resources for financial counsel and guidance are available to members of our ministry team?

The Biblical Design for Life in Ministry

VOCATIONAL WELLNESS

In One Word: HUMILITY

(The Fruit of the Spirit is GENTLENESS)

My joyful following of God's call into kingdom service, utilizing the gifts he has imparted in a spirit of GENTLENESS (Gal. 5:23) and servanthood.

A Word from Ephesians 4:11-12

It was he who gave some to be apostles, some to be prophets, some to be evangelists, and some to be pastors and teachers, to prepare God's people *for works of service,* so that the body of Christ may be built up.

Summary Marker of Vocational Wellness

As I grow in God's grace of Vocational GENTLENESS,
I am finding joy in HUMILITY as I serve through my calling and gifts.

The JOY of Life in Ministry is interrupted when unreasonable expectations and overfunctioning contribute to frustration and hindered ministry efforts.

Vocational Wellness is the healing touch of Christ restoring the joy of living in Vocational Humility by the Holy Spirit's gift of Gentleness.

Growth in the Vocational life is learning to identify my gifts and passions and those of others so that together we are learning to serve in the power of the Spirit.

Vocational Wellness in Churches happens when Pastor and other professional church workers are serving in unity and cooperation with all leaders and members of the congregation.

Additional Scriptures: 1 Corinthians 12; Romans 12; 1 Peter 4:7-11; 1 Timothy 3-4, 6; Matthew 25:14-30.

Biblical examples of Vocational Wellness: Elijah (1 Kings 19); Stephen (Acts 6); Timothy (1&2 Timothy); Matthew 25.

Narrative Description of Vocational Wellness

Following his mountaintop experience and the great victory over Baal's prophets, Elijah crashed. He ran for his life then fell down exhausted, discouraged and lonely. It's a story of church worker burnout that is repeated far too often in our own time. God's intention for people in ministry and their families is the gift of joy. The privilege of serving as bearers of the good news should be cause for celebration, seeing firsthand the work of the Spirit through the Word. Most professional church workers, however, have at some point experienced the anxieties of the ministry life that can diminish the joy.

Healthy, mature church workers are regularly humbled by their calling, and also by their inadequacy for the task. Healthy, mature church members recognize the unique stresses that are inherent in a life of Christian ministry. Together, church workers and church members can strive to create an environment for ministry where those called into Christian ministry will be continually renewed and refreshed in Christ, at their very best, to the benefit of all they serve.

Vocational wellness for church workers and for every disciple of Christ is found when the joy of ministry predominates over the stresses and burdens. Some of the things that contribute to joy in ministry are a common vision and passion for the Lord's work; a vibrant spiritual life; mutual care and concern for one another; Christ-centered conflict resolution; and appropriate, reasonable expectations of one another.

God gave Elijah the gift of a friend and the promise that he was not alone. The partnership between church workers and church members can be a most beautiful expression of community.

PHYSICAL WELLNESS

In One Word: VITALITY
(The Fruit of the Spirit is SELF-CONTROL)

My life by the Spirit's gift of SELF-CONTROL (Gal. 5:23) over the unhealthy passions of the body for the sake my calling to serve family, church and community.

A Word from Ephesians 4:17-20

So I tell you this, and insist on it in the Lord, that you must no longer live as the Gentiles do, in the futility of their thinking. They are darkened in their understanding and separated from the life of God because of the ignorance that is in them due to the hardening of their hearts. Having lost all sensitivity, they have given themselves over to sensuality so as to indulge in every kind of impurity, with a continual lust for more. You, however, did not come to know Christ that way.

Summary Marker of Physical Wellness

As I grow in God's grace of Physical SELF-CONTROL,
I am finding joy in the VITALITY that flows from practicing healthy choices.

The JOY of Life in Ministry is interrupted when following the appetites of the flesh that harm the wellbeing of the body hinders the vitality that God has given and leaves me less capable of being an instrument of his goodness.

Physical Wellness is the healing touch of Christ restoring the joy of living in Physical Vitality, by the Holy Spirit's gift of Self-Control.

Growth in the Physical life is learning to discover the benefits of stress management, proper nutrition, appropriate exercise, adequate rest, and regular health screenings for physical wellbeing.

Physical Wellness in Churches happens when the local body of Christ fosters the physical health of young and old in the congregation.

Additional Scriptures: 1 Kings 19; Leviticus 11; Daniel 1; 1 Corinthians 6:12-20; Romans 6-7

Biblical examples of Physical Wellness: Jesus (Mark 4:38, 6:31); Elijah (1 Kings 19); Daniel (Daniel 1)

Narrative Description of Physical Wellness

Daniel and his friends had work to do. As God's people in a foreign land, they wanted to give their best witness to the Lord, and their vigor and vitality for their daily tasks was part of that witness. The fruit of the Spirit is self-control. Daniel sought a healthy diet for a healthy body so he would be ready and able to respond to the Lord's call. He was, and he did!

The healing ministry of Jesus continues in our congregations. In his providential care, God has allowed infirmity and disability to fall to many of His children. The body of Christ surrounds these servants of Christ with care and provision for their every need. In our day, because of the neglect of healthy practices like nutrition, exercise and rest, many of us bring weakness and disease upon ourselves. The levels of many stress related illnesses are higher among clergy than they are in the general population.

Our churches are in an ideal position to teach the Lord's people to honor God in the care of their bodies. God created these bodies of ours and redeemed them by the blood of our incarnate Savior. And we'll spend eternity in glorious bodies, for we believe in the resurrection of the body.

We sing, "Take my hands and let them move at the impulse of Thy love" (LSB 783). Jesus said that the washing of feet was done as an example for us, that we would show our love in deeds of service. When our bodies are as healthy and fit as they can be, we are, like Daniel, ready and able to respond to the Lord's call to serve.

FINANCIAL WELLNESS

In One Word: GENEROSITY
(The Fruit of the Spirit is FAITHFULNESS)

My confident trust in God's provision that leads to FAITHFULNESS (Gal. 5:22) to the call to share his material blessings for the advancement of his Kingdom.

A Word from Ephesians 4:21-24

He who has been stealing must steal no longer, but must work, doing something useful with his own hands, that he may have something to *share with those in need.*

Summary Marker of Financial Wellness

As I grow in God's grace of Financial FAITHFULNESS,
I am finding joy in GENEROSITY, sharing with others as I have been blessed.

The JOY of Life in Ministry is interrupted when, like the Rich Fool, hoarding the good gifts of God disrupts his intention that all would be blessed through the abundance we share.

Financial Wellness is the healing touch of Christ restoring the joy of living in Financial Generosity, by the Holy Spirit's gift of Faithfulness.

Growth in the Financial life is learning to grow day by day in the grace of trusting, faithful generosity.

Financial Wellness in Churches happens when the local body of Christ knows that God's provision is assured, so we freely offer what is already his.

Additional Scriptures: 2 Corinthians 8-9; Luke 12:13-21; 1 Chronicles 29:1-20; 1 Timothy 6:3-10.

Biblical examples of Financial Wellness: Widow's Mite (Luke 21:1-4); Macedonian Christians (2 Corinthians 8); The Philippian Church (Philippians 4).

Narrative Description of Financial Wellness

When Jesus said, "Eat, drink and be merry" it was spoken as a horribly bad example! The Rich Fool who said it died that night and left his wealth behind (see Luke 12:13-21). God did not design us to be reservoirs of his blessing, storing up wealth for our own selfish use. He designed us to be rivers of generosity.

Lutheran Women in Mission have changed the world through their generosity, following the example of the poor widow who shared her last two small coins. Professional church workers are both supported by such generosity, and serve as examples of such sacrificial, first-fruits giving. Teaching the whole counsel of God, including the biblical principles of stewardship and contentment, encourages a lifestyle of generous giving. The culture that surrounds us measures a person's value by the size of their bank account and the abundance of their material goods, but we know that our worth is not measured by gold or silver, but the precious blood of Jesus Christ.

Financially healthy congregations make it possible for their called workers to serve with joy and gladness, free of financial worries. Leaders of healthy congregations annually study the district's suggested salary guidelines for workers, found on the district website, and do their best to meet the guidelines. Many congregations establish a salary floor, a percentage of the guidelines below which salaries must not fall.

And healthy congregations and their workers together give God thanks and praise for his faithfulness and abundant provision for all of their needs.

MINISTRY TEAM CONVERSATION ON THE "LIFE IN COMMUNITY" WELLNESS ASSESSMENT

Discuss together the "Markers of Wellbeing" as they apply to your Ministry Team's corporate wellness.

Summary Marker of Vocational Wellness

As I grow in God's grace of Vocational GENTLENESS,
I am finding joy in HUMILITY as I serve through my calling and gifts.

Summary Marker of Physical Wellness

As I grow in God's grace of Physical SELF-CONTROL,
I am finding joy in the VITALITY that flows from practicing healthy choices.

Summary Marker of Financial Wellness

As I grow in God's grace of Financial FAITHFULNESS,
I am finding joy in GENEROSITY, sharing with others as I have been blessed.

9

Which Makes Daily Healing Essential

A MAN CRIPPLED FROM BIRTH met Peter and John as they went through the Beautiful Gate to the Jerusalem Temple, and something wonderful happened: he was saved. Or he was healed. And saved. It was one or the other, either saved or healed. Or it might have been both. The word that Luke used to describe what happened to the man in Acts chapter 4 leaves us wondering a little bit what exactly he experienced, salvation or healing.

The language of our faith is always in danger of becoming worn thin. Some of the words we use, like "saved" and "healed" have been bandied about for so long and we've heard them so often that they are in danger of losing their meaning. These words are our treasure, especially the metaphors for salvation, ("salvation" itself being one of those), and maybe "saved" is a word that's been worn thin more than any of the others. It's the job of preachers to keep these words alive, vibrant and meaningful, so let me give it a try.

According to the New International Version, Peter and John said that they were on trial for "an act of kindness shown to a cripple and [we] are asked how he was healed" (Acts 4:9, emphasis added). The Greek word for healed here is "sōdzō," the exact same word used in verse 12, "Salvation is found in no one else, for there is no other name under heaven given to men by which we must be saved." Saved? Healed? Why the confusion? I went straight to Kittel's Theological Dictionary of the New Testament and looked up "sōdzō." I discovered that "sōdzō," which is most commonly translated either "healed" or "saved," in Acts 4 is "perhaps deliberately ambiguous."[41] What a great expression: perhaps deliberately ambiguous! It's not a choice between saved and healed. "Sōdzō" is what Jesus does whenever his gifts of grace are received by faith. Jesus saves. Jesus heals.

The gospel record tells of Jesus moving throughout Galilee, healing and proclaiming the reign of God over sin, death and the devil. In the healing/saving of the paralyzed man in Mark 2, Jesus made it clear that the restoration of broken humanity, both the forgiveness of sin and the removal of the debilitating effects of sin, is all of one piece. "Which is easier: to say to the paralytic, 'Your sins are forgiven,' or to say, 'Get up, take your mat and walk?'" (Mark 2:9). Which is easier, to save or to heal? Where sin is forgiven, the grip of sin loses its hold. Salvation is healing. Healing is a gospel metaphor that we'd like to keep alive and fresh with the full nuanced understanding of God's lifelong work in the lives of his children, as the scriptures so often affirm. "He heals the brokenhearted and binds up their wounds" (Psalm 147:3). [42] "Healing" is a beautiful way to describe what Elijah experienced through the gracious work of God following his collapse under the broom tree. "Healing" describes the work of God in the lives of all who follow Christ.

I guess by now you can see where Lesson Nine fits on the journey to wellness and joy in ministry. Ministry is great, but hard, because it's the way of the cross and overwhelmed is a way of life so don't try this alone. Joy fuels ministry, but ministry threatens the joy of life with God and life in community and life in ministry, which makes daily healing essential for professional church workers.

RESTORATION OF A FALLEN AND BROKEN WORLD

The gospel metaphor of healing is pervasive throughout the scriptures. In Numbers 21 people of faith are rescued from the viper's bite[43]. In Leviticus 13-14 the priests affirm the healing work of God by welcoming the healed back into the community. In 1 Kings 17 Elijah raised the widow's son. In 2 Kings 5 Elisha takes the redemptive/healing work of God international as Naaman the Aramean is healed from leprosy. In the New Testament Gospel of Mark there are more miraculous healings recorded than in the entire Old Testament! It's the work of God that leads his people to sing, "Praise the Lord, O my soul, and forget not all his benefits—who forgives all your sins and heals all your diseases"(Psalm 103:2-3).

I'll readily agree that much of what is termed "Christian healing" is not really healing at all and hardly Christian, but if you are called into a church work career, you're called to carry on the healing ministry of Jesus. "Healing ministry" is a term that needs reclaiming and clarification. Care for the physical needs of people is part of it. Most hospitals in America were established by Christian ministries. We believe in the power of God to work physical miracles of healing, as a part of his work of greater healing by the gospel. That proclamation of the gospel brings healing beyond the miraculous deliverance from bodily ills. It touches every aspect of life.

Allow me to be blunt: professional church workers can't bring gifts of God to others that they have not first experienced in their own lives. It's crucial that church workers wrap their head around this concept: Jesus uses our own experiences of healing, our own scars, as part of his plan to advance the kingdom. We share Christ not from our position of perfection, but from our place as those who have first, often, and daily received

> Jesus uses our own experiences of healing, our own scars, as part of his plan to advance the kingdom.

his healing grace. Paul described the life of a church worker explicitly and graphically: "We are hard pressed on every side, but not crushed; perplexed, but not in despair; persecuted, but not abandoned; struck down, but not destroyed. We always carry around in our body the death of Jesus, so that the life of Jesus may also be revealed in our body. For we who are alive are always being given over to death for Jesus' sake, so that his life may be revealed in our mortal body" (2 Corinthians 4:8-11).

The immortal life of Christ is on display in our mortality, in these frail, weak, broken, and yet healed and mended, lives of ours. Do you remember how this passage from 2 Corinthians 4 began? "But we have this treasure in jars of clay to show that this all-surpassing power is from God and not from us." The people who look to us for good news from God do not need superheroes. They need to see jars of clay; lumpy, leaky, cracked pots put together again by a power greater than we ourselves, the power of Christ. Broken and in need of healing is a good place to be, because only the lowly are able to rejoice in the gift of grace and sing, "Praise the Lord, O my soul, and forget not all his benefits—who forgives all your sins and heals all your diseases" (Psalm 103:2-3).

It's why the 2,000 year long story of the advancement of the kingdom is written in the blood, sweat, and tears of the Lord's kingdom workers. It's why God in his wisdom allowed the deaths of the martyrs; in them the resurrection of Christ was revealed, and the martyrs were healed as they gained the life everlasting. It's why Paul could say that his thorn in the flesh served to advance the gospel, for the power of Christ was on display in his weakness (see 2 Corinthians 12:7-10). In his classic work, "The Wounded Healer," Henri Nouwen lifts up the critical importance of leading others by our own personal experience of restoration and healing. "The great illusion of leadership is to think that [a person] can be led out of the desert by someone who has never been there."[44]

The people we seek to lead to the saving/healing grace of Jesus are constantly assessing our integrity, testing the truth of what we proclaim. When we speak of God's work in the gospel, it's only natural for our listeners to be asking, "Oh, really?" They want to know if we know what we're talking about; if we really know what we're professing. Walther said it like this: "A [church worker] who has not been through this experience is a sound without meaning, a sounding brass and a tinkling cymbal. But [someone] who has personally passed through this experience can really speak from the heart, and what he says will go into the hearts of his hearers."[45] In a certain sense, everything we share about the saving/healing power of Christ is laced through with our own experience of that power, and the words that Nouwen used: "been there." First, we're healed; then we're healers.

The theme of this chapter is that those who carry on the healing ministry of Jesus do that work best from a deep understanding of the Lord's gift of healing in their own lives. The "been there" for church workers is both "been to the desert" and "been to the healing fountain of grace." It's the lesson of the oxygen mask on the airliner. In order to be of use to those who depend on us, we first must breathe deeply ourselves. Those who feed others have first known what hunger is, but have tasted the banquet themselves. Those who bear the healing touch have felt both the pain of brokenness and the embrace of grace in their own lives.

The "healing" metaphor works well for us at Grace Place Wellness, partly because it rings true to the experience of Dr. Eckrich in his medical practice and in his restorative work with so many church workers over the years, but also because it speaks to the reality of our daily need for the gospel of Christ. As we journey by faith, we get whacked every day spiritually, physically and emotionally. Lesson Nine, "Daily healing is essential," is a reminder that as we begin each day's labors anew, we are desperately in need of healing from yesterday's wounds. And just as our Creator is constantly at work replenishing and restoring our bodies by his gifts of nutrition and rest, he is always at work restoring us by his grace and love, strengthening us for the next day's calling.

Our grandparents never discarded anything, they just mended what was broken and put it back into use. God is a mender. He found Elijah on the junk heap, restored him by the Word of hope, and sent him back into ministry. The perceptive church worker is continually aware of those worn through spots, the places in their lives where the handle has broken off or the wiring has become frayed or the hose has sprung a leak. Recognizing how the wear and tear of ministry has left them diminished, they know where to go to find repair for their torn relationships, for their wounded psyches and for their exhausted bodies: the cross and empty tomb of Jesus Christ.

SUBSTANTIAL HEALING

I'm not suggesting that we will ever in this life experience perfect healing. This side of glory we continue to bear the cross of our physical, emotional, financial and vocational scars, but the healing power of the gospel is real. It's significant. It is life-changing. I like Francis Schaeffer's adjective for the healing work of the gospel as we journey by faith. He calls it "substantial" healing. That's the kind of healing we're talking about in Lesson Nine, daily renewal in the grace of Christ that is not yet perfect, but substantial, fueling us with the gift of joy. We have a God-instilled yearning for the complete and perfect ideal, total restoration to the Garden of Eden, but the fulfillment of that dream is not our lot while still on our way to heaven. But neither are we without hope or without the healing touch of the gospel of grace. Schaeffer first talks about the relational aspect of this substantial, but not yet perfect, healing.

"The alternatives are not between being perfect or being nothing. Just as people smash marriages because they are looking for what is romantically and sexually perfect and in this poor world do not find it, so human beings often smash what could have been possible in a true church or true Christian group. It is not just the 'they' involved who are not yet perfect, but the 'I' is not yet perfect either. In the absence of present perfection, Christians are to help each other on to increasingly substantial healing on the basis of the finished work of Christ. This is our calling."[46]

In the context of our conversation, I take Schaeffer's reference to the "they" and the "I" to mean the people we serve and their called servants. Church workers and congregations are engaged in the lifelong cooperative effort to help each other increasingly experience the substantial healing that Jesus brings to every aspect of life.

Christ's healing work has an impact on the deepest parts of our being; never complete in this earthly life, but again, substantial.

"This also does not mean that we will be perfect in this life psychologically any more than we are physically. But thank God, now I can move; I am no longer running on ice, that is the difference. It does not need to be the old, endless circle. It is not any longer the dog chasing his tail. The light is let in. Things are orientated, and I can move as a whole man, with all the rationality I possess utterly in place. I will not expect to be perfect. I will wait for the second coming of Jesus Christ and the resurrection of the body, to be perfect morally, physically, and psychologically; but there now can be a substantive overcoming of this psychological division in the present life on the basis of Christ's finished work.

> **During this time of bearing the cross, however, the work of the Holy Spirit to bring healing in our lives is never finished.**

It will not be perfect, but it can be real and substantial. Let us be clear about this. All men since the fall have had some psychological problems. It is utter nonsense, a romanticism that has nothing to do with biblical Christianity, to say that a Christian never has a psychological problem. All men have psychological problems. They differ in degree and they differ in kind, but since the fall all men have more or less a problem psychologically. And dealing with this, too, is a part of the present aspect of the gospel and of the finished work of Christ on Calvary's cross."[47]

The New Testament confirms over and over again that the redemptive work of Christ was completed on the cross, at the resurrection and at his ascension to the throne of glory. All that is necessary for the forgiveness of sins and entrance into God's eternal kingdom is finished, accomplished perfectly, once and for all and for all time. There is nothing left to be done.

During this time of bearing the cross, however, the work of the Holy Spirit to bring healing in our lives is never finished.

The first eight lessons on the wellness journey have not been easy, but we're nearing the end, and it's time for more hopeful news. At Grace Place Wellness Ministries, we believe that despite our brokenness, the healing ministry of Jesus continues still today, and so Lesson Nine on the journey to wellness, "Daily healing is essential," is a call to seek and to welcome the healing/saving work of Christ in our own lives every single day. A few unusual individuals will skip quickly through Lessons One through Eight because they know intuitively and learned early on that they will daily need to experience the healing work of the Spirit. Most of us learned it the hard way by the long, slow process of digesting the previous eight steps on the journey. Sadly, many ministers never get this far in the journey toward self-care and wellness.

At Grace Place Wellness Ministries we define wellness as "Christ's healing love restoring the joy of receiving God's grace, living in community with others, and serving through our vocations." The healing touch of Christ is the cure for the disease we examined in Lessons Six, Seven and Eight.

So what would the healing touch of Christ look like for a church worker who had lost the Spirit's gift of joy?

When life with God begins to feel like a journey through the wilderness, the healing touch of Christ restores the joy of salvation. The Holy Spirit, working through the living Word of God fills heart and soul with words of promise, hope, forgiveness and grace and renews the baptismal joy of living as a child of the heavenly Father.

When life in community with others at home, at church or in the ministry team becomes clouded with the bad atmosphere of factions, dissension and hurt feelings, the healing touch of Christ restores the joy of Christian unity for which we were created. By confessing our sins to God and to one another, and affirming his healing grace to each other, Satan runs, harmony and love are restored, and the joy of life together returns.

When life in ministry becomes just a job, and when thoughts of leaving the call to gospel service begin to creep in, the healing touch of Christ renews the vision for the highest calling on earth. Eyes of faith are opened to see that in every ministration of the Word of Christ, God himself is at work transforming lives for time and for eternity. The joy of being used as the humble instruments of God for the salvation of the world lifts hearts and spirits, and, like Elijah and the countless servants of the gospel before us, we engage once again in the joy of the Lord.

THE HEALING POWER OF THE GOSPEL

How about you? When you find yourself under the broom tree, (or sidling up next to it), do you find the healing touch of Jesus that restores the joy of Life with God, the joy of Life in Community and the joy of Life in Ministry? Do you receive the gifts of God that are needed to bring you substantial healing, and do you hear the voice of the Lord telling you, as he told Elijah, "Go back the way you came"?

Find your joy in the promise of a loving Father who provides all that you need, every gift of body, mind and spirit necessary to continue on in your calling. Luther concluded his description of God's providential care with a call to continued service: "For all which it is my duty to thank and praise, serve and obey him."[48]

Find your joy in the gift of a Savior, who humbled himself and became a servant of the world by offering his life, and who rose again and has come to you with a call to follow. He is still calling, and he is still present with you every day to heal and restore you from yesterday's hurts. His continued work of touching your life for healing is to enable you to continue his work of healing ministry. Luther said it this way, "...that I may be his own and live under him in his kingdom and serve him in everlasting righteousness, innocence and blessedness."[49]

> His continued work of touching your life for healing is to enable you to continue his work of healing ministry.

Find your joy in the outpouring of the Holy Spirit in your life, who, Luther reminds us, "...has called me by the gospel, [and] enlightened me with his gifts."[50] As long as you have life and breath, find joy in knowing that the Lord himself fills you with gifts for service in his kingdom.

Cracked pots of clay that we are, church workers don't always feel adequate for the calling, for the daily and weekly tasks of ministry. Regardless of how you might feel, the healing work of Christ makes you worthy and prepares you for the calling. That's why, as Lesson Nine reminds us, "Daily healing is essential."

DAILY HEALING

Daily healing is essential for those carrying the burdens of ministry, and God's Means of Grace are his divinely instituted delivery system for the healing that we need. Jesus remains present among the gathered church through his gifts of Word and Sacrament. Through these gifts we receive wholeness as life with God is restored, as life in community is made whole again and as life in service is re-launched.

Baptism is a gift for your healing. In God's gracious anointing and claim on your life, you can always know that your identity as his child and servant is sure and secure.

The celebration of The Lord's Supper is a gift for your healing in body and soul. Jesus himself comes in this blessed gift to forgive, renew and strengthen you for your service.

Daily forgiveness at the foot of the cross is a gift for your healing. When you daily place the failures and regrets of yesterday at his feet, as he wipes them away by grace, you're given a new beginning.

Prayer is certainly a gift for our healing. You are never alone in your ministry. Humbly calling out to God for strength is your act of faith that your Father in heaven honors and truly hears.

And, of course, the Word of God is a healing force in the lives of all touched by its gifts of grace. To those who humbly cry to the Lord for help, "He sent forth his word and healed them; he rescued them from the grave" (Psalm 107:20). Ministers of the gospel proclaim the message of hope and comfort because it saves and heals. We know it's true because we ourselves run to that binding, restoring message of forgiveness, hope and joy every day. Baptismal renewal, the reception of the Lord's body and blood, absolution and prayer all find their therapeutic power in the abiding promises of God's mercy upon his children.

As we've mentioned before, the healing ministry of professional church workers to their people is to be mutual. The congregational community is called to offer care, nurture and healing ministry to all of its members, including those who lead the ministry, their professional church workers. What a joy and comfort it is for ministers and members to become together a community of healing, to renew their baptismal blessings together, to gather together at the table and break from one loaf together and to announce the words of forgiveness and grace to one another! Some congregations fulfill their responsibility to care for their called workers better than others, but it remains the responsibility of all professional church workers to develop a plan and disciplines for their own self-care to ensure that they are experiencing the daily healing touch of Christ in their own lives.

In the next chapter I'll introduce you to the wellness model that has been a blessing to thousands of professional church workers and their families for more than two decades, a model to guide you to seek and to find the Lord's healing touch every day, the healing touch that restores the joy of Life with God, Life in Community and Life in Ministry.

Before I do, make some time soon to carefully work through Not Finished Yet and then the material that follows right after, the Grace Place Wellness Assessment Inventory. It's designed to help you reflect on what you've learned in the first Nine Lessons and possibly identify that aspect of wellness where you are most in need of the Lord's healing touch of grace to restore to you the gift of his own joy!

NOT FINISHED YET!

Take a few minutes to consider whether Lesson Nine, "Daily healing is essential" is a lesson about ministry that you've taken to heart.

» What did you read in this chapter that resonates most deeply? What made you say to yourself, "That's really true!"?

» How would you phrase Lesson Nine differently?

» What did Darrell not discuss in this chapter that really could have been mentioned?

» If this is a lesson you've already learned from your own experience, when did you first discover that it was true?

» What needs your further contemplation before moving on to the next chapter?

MINISTRY TEAM CONVERSATION STARTERS
FOR LESSON NINE

» In what ways have you experienced hurt and brokenness because of your life in ministry, Spiritually, Relationally, and Vocationally?

» How have you experienced the healing grace of Christ in your life?

» How would you like to see your ministry team become more of a healing community for one another?

Assessing Personal Wellness

PART 1: LIFE WITH GOD

Review the comments on Baptismal and Spiritual brokenness and wellness in Lesson 6, "Ministry Threatens the Joy of Life with God," and also the descriptions of biblical wellness given at the end of Lesson 6.1.

What forces threatening a church worker's Baptismal and Spiritual Wellness resonate with you? How have you experienced that brokenness in your own life?

Baptismal Wellness

Rate each of the following:

Almost Never   **1**   **2**   **3**   **4**   **5**   **6**   *Almost Always*

____ The Spirit faithfully gives me the joy of knowing the unconditional love of Jesus.

____ I find confidence, comfort and security in my identity as God's child.

____ I'm learning to put off the old self and rise to new life daily (Eph. 4:21-24).

Where do you fall on the Healthy/Unhealthy scale?

HEALTHY							UNHEALTHY
New creation	6	5	4	3	2	1	Old nature
Christ in me	6	5	4	3	2	1	Me in me
Loved	6	5	4	3	2	1	Lost
Freedom	6	5	4	3	2	1	Stuck
Hope	6	5	4	3	2	1	Despair
Butterfly	6	5	4	3	2	1	Caterpillar
Belonging	6	5	4	3	2	1	Loneliness

____ **Total Baptismal**

Make some notes on your Baptismal Wellness here.

»   In what circumstances do you exhibit Baptismal resilience?

»   What makes you feel vulnerable? What makes you hurt?

Spiritual Wellness

Rate each of the following:

Almost Never   **1**   **2**   **3**   **4**   **5**   **6**   *Almost Always*

____ The Spirit faithfully gives me the joy of God imparting his goodness to me.

____ By my daily and weekly disciplines, I exhibit my receptivity to God's gifts of grace.

____ God is not finished, but I am becoming mature, growing in faith and love (Eph. 4:13-16).

Where do you fall on the Healthy/Unhealthy scale?

HEALTHY							UNHEALTHY
Fullness	6	5	4	3	2	1	Emptiness
Hungry/Thirsty	6	5	4	3	2	1	Satisfied
Maturing	6	5	4	3	2	1	Immature
Formation	6	5	4	3	2	1	Information
Growth	6	5	4	3	2	1	Stagnation
Devotion	6	5	4	3	2	1	Busy-ness
Grounded	6	5	4	3	2	1	Tossed

____ Total Spiritual

Make some notes on your Spiritual Wellness here.

» In what circumstances do you exhibit Spiritual resilience?

» What makes you feel vulnerable? What makes you hurt?

PART 2: LIFE IN COMMUNITY

Review the comments on Relational, Intellectual and Emotional brokenness and wellness in Lesson 7, "Ministry Threatens the Joy of Life in Community," and also the descriptions of biblical wellness given at the end of Lesson 7.1.

What forces threatening a church worker's Relational, Intellectual and Emotional Wellness resonate with you? How have you experienced that brokenness in your own life?

Relational Wellness

Rate each of the following:

Almost Never   **1**   **2**   **3**   **4**   **5**   **6**   *Almost Always*

____ The Spirit faithfully gives me the joy of showing patience toward others.

____ My relationships reflect the Spirit's gift of unity, intrinsic to the body of Christ.

____ I am growing more humble, gentle, patient and loving (Eph. 4:2-6).

Where do you fall on the Healthy/Unhealthy scale?

HEALTHY							UNHEALTHY
Respect	6	5	4	3	2	1	Contempt
Patience	6	5	4	3	2	1	Impatience
Loyalty	6	5	4	3	2	1	Treachery
Synergy	6	5	4	3	2	1	Division
Cleaving	6	5	4	3	2	1	Leaving
Servanthood	6	5	4	3	2	1	Selfishness
Trust	6	5	4	3	2	1	Suspicion

___ Total Relational

Make some notes on your Relational Wellness here.

» In what circumstances do you exhibit Relational resilience?

» What makes you feel vulnerable? What makes you hurt?

Intellectual Wellness

Rate each of the following:

Almost Never   **1**   **2**   **3**   **4**   **5**   **6**   *Almost Always*

____ The Spirit faithfully gives me the joy of kindness and sincere listening.

____ I display a healthy curiosity about what I might learn from the wisdom of others.

____ I am learning to speak only truthful words that will build up those who hear (Eph. 4:25, 29).

Where do you fall on the Healthy/Unhealthy scale?

HEALTHY							**UNHEALTHY**
Open	6	5	4	3	2	1	Closed
Honesty	6	5	4	3	2	1	Deception
Sharing	6	5	4	3	2	1	Hiding
Discovery	6	5	4	3	2	1	Ignorance
Curiosity	6	5	4	3	2	1	Prejudice
Compassion	6	5	4	3	2	1	Indifference
Listening	6	5	4	3	2	1	Attributing

___ **Total Intellectual**

Make some notes on your Intellectual Wellness here.

» In what circumstances do you exhibit Intellectual resilience?

» What makes you feel vulnerable? What makes you hurt?

Emotional Wellbeing

Rate each of the following:

Almost Never   **1   2   3   4   5   6**   *Almost Always*

____ The Spirit faithfully gives me the joy of peace-filled relationships.

____ My relationships in family and church are characterized by harmony.

____ I am growing in the graces of kindness, compassion and forgiveness (Eph. 4:26-32).

Where do you fall on the Healthy/Unhealthy scale?

HEALTHY							UNHEALTHY
Sunny	6	5	4	3	2	1	Stormy
Light Mood	6	5	4	3	2	1	Dark Mood
Joyful	6	5	4	3	2	1	Serious
Harmony	6	5	4	3	2	1	Conflict
Grace	6	5	4	3	2	1	Grudges
Good Feelings	6	5	4	3	2	1	Hurt Feelings
Confession	6	5	4	3	2	1	Blame

___ **Total Emotional**

Make some notes on your Emotional Wellness here.

»   In what circumstances do you exhibit Emotional resilience?

»   What makes you feel vulnerable? What makes you hurt?

PART 3: LIFE IN MINISTRY

Review the comments on Vocational, Physical and Financial brokenness and wellness in Lesson 8, "Ministry Threatens the Joy of Life in Ministry," and also the descriptions of biblical wellness given at the end of Lesson 8.1.

What forces threatening a church worker's Vocational, Physical and Financial Wellness resonate with you? How have you experienced that brokenness in your own life?

Vocational Wellbeing

Rate each of the following:

Almost Never   **1**   **2**   **3**   **4**   **5**   **6**   *Almost Always*

____ The Spirit faithfully gives me the joy of serving others in a spirit of gentleness.

____ God's call to a life of service is an ever-increasing source of humility.

____ I am often able to recognize ways that God uses me to build up the body of Christ (Eph. 4:11-12).

Where do you fall on the Healthy/Unhealthy scale?

HEALTHY							UNHEALTHY
Passion-driven	6	5	4	3	2	1	Job Description driven
Spirit-led	6	5	4	3	2	1	Ego-led
Joyful	6	5	4	3	2	1	Burdensome
Boundaries	6	5	4	3	2	1	Overfunctioning
Energized	6	5	4	3	2	1	Burnt out
Gitta	6	5	4	3	2	1	Gotta
Servant	6	5	4	3	2	1	Authority

____ Total Vocational

Make some notes on your Vocational Wellness here.

»   In what circumstances do you exhibit Vocational resilience?

»   What makes you feel vulnerable? What makes you hurt?

Physical Wellbeing

Rate each of the following:

Almost Never   **1**   **2**   **3**   **4**   **5**   **6**   *Almost Always*

____ The Spirit faithfully gives me the joy of self-control as the flesh's passions are subdued.

____ My physical health choices result in vitality for service to God, family and church.

____ While always present, my physical passions and desires do not control me (Eph. 4:17-20).

Where do you fall on the Healthy/Unhealthy scale?

HEALTHY							UNHEALTHY
Rested	6	5	4	3	2	1	Exhausted
Eustress	6	5	4	3	2	1	Distress
Energy	6	5	4	3	2	1	Lethargy
Natural food	6	5	4	3	2	1	Processed food
Self-control	6	5	4	3	2	1	Lust
Active	6	5	4	3	2	1	Sedentary
Moderation	6	5	4	3	2	1	Indulgence

____ **Total Physical**

Make some notes on your Physical Wellness here.

» In what circumstances do you exhibit Physical resilience?

» What makes you feel vulnerable? What makes you hurt?

Financial Wellbeing

Rate each of the following:

Almost Never   **1   2   3   4   5   6**   *Almost Always*

____ The Spirit faithfully gives me the joy of faithfulness in my stewardship of resources.

____ I respond appropriately to opportunities to show generosity.

____ I remember that I am provided for abundantly so I can share with those in need (Eph. 4:28).

Where do you fall on the Healthy/Unhealthy scale?

HEALTHY							**UNHEALTHY**
Gratitude	6	5	4	3	2	1	Ingratitude
Sacrifice	6	5	4	3	2	1	Hoard
Contentment	6	5	4	3	2	1	Desire
Sharing	6	5	4	3	2	1	Accumulating
Planning	6	5	4	3	2	1	Chance
Trust	6	5	4	3	2	1	Fear
Generosity	6	5	4	3	2	1	Selfishness

____ Total Financial

Make some notes on your Financial Wellness here.

»   In what circumstances do you exhibit Financial resilience?

»   What makes you feel vulnerable? What makes you hurt?

Where to Begin: Assessing Wellness

Grace Place Wellness Ministries has designed a workbook to help you develop an intentional growth plan. The *Reclaiming the Joy of Ministry* Workbook Series is a self-directed workshop to help you move to the next part of your wellness journey beginning with that aspect of wellness where the Spirit's gift of joy is most significantly depleted. The workbooks, one for each of the aspects of wellness on the Wellness Wheel, are described in greater detail in the Appendix following the next chapter and are available through our website **GracePlaceWellness.org**.

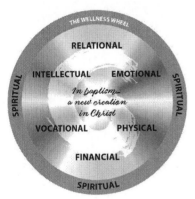

What does the above exercise indicate may be the aspect of your wellness from the Wellness Wheel that most needs the healing touch of Christ in your life right now?

Do the assessment tools above match up with your own experience in recent months, affirming what you have sensed about your wellbeing?

If not, where do you feel you are currently experiencing the greatest need?

List here, in order of priority, which three aspects of wellness need your attention. We strongly encourage you to address the most critical need first, returning for work in the other areas only after you have experienced substantial healing in your first priority.

My areas of growth:

Choose one for immediate attention:

Life with God   ____ Baptismal   ____ Spiritual

Life in Community   ____ Relational   ____ Intellectual ____ Emotional

Life in Ministry   ____ Vocational   ____ Physical   ____ Financial

Choose one for future consideration (after addressing the above):

Life with God   ____ Baptismal   ____ Spiritual

Life in Community   ____ Relational   ____ Intellectual ____ Emotional

Life in Ministry   ____ Vocational   ____ Physical   ____ Financial

Choose one for eventual consideration (after addressing both of the above):

Life with God   ____ Baptismal   ____ Spiritual

Life in Community   ____ Relational   ____ Intellectual ____ Emotional

Life in Ministry   ____ Vocational   ____ Physical   ____ Financial

LESSON 9.2

Assessing Ministry Team Wellness

Now complete the Assessment, this time focusing not on your own personal wellness, but focusing on the wellness exhibited in your life and work together as a ministry team.

PART 1: LIFE WITH GOD

Review the comments on Baptismal and Spiritual brokenness and wellness in Lesson 6, "Ministry Threatens the Joy of Life with God," and also the descriptions of biblical wellness given at the end of Lesson 6.1.

What forces threatening your team's Baptismal and Spiritual Wellness resonate with you? How have you experienced that brokenness in your life together in ministry?

Baptismal Wellness

Rate each of the following:

Almost Never   **1**   **2**   **3**   **4**   **5**   **6**   *Almost Always*

____ The Spirit faithfully gives us the joy of knowing the unconditional love of Jesus.

____ We find confidence, comfort and security in our identity as God's children.

____ We're learning to put off the old self and rise to new life daily (Eph. 4:21-24).

Where does your team fall on the Healthy/Unhealthy scale?

HEALTHY							UNHEALTHY
New creation	6	5	4	3	2	1	Old nature
Christ in me	6	5	4	3	2	1	Me in me
Loved	6	5	4	3	2	1	Lost
Freedom	6	5	4	3	2	1	Stuck
Hope	6	5	4	3	2	1	Despair
Butterfly	6	5	4	3	2	1	Caterpillar
Belonging	6	5	4	3	2	1	Loneliness

____ Total Baptismal

Make some notes on your team's Baptismal Wellness here.

» In what circumstances does your team exhibit Baptismal resilience?

» What makes you feel vulnerable? What makes you hurt?

Spiritual Wellness

Rate each of the following:

Almost Never   **1**   **2**   **3**   **4**   **5**   **6**   *Almost Always*

____ The Spirit faithfully gives us the joy of God imparting his goodness to us.

____ By our daily and weekly disciplines, we exhibit our receptivity to God's gifts of grace.

____ God is not finished, but we are becoming mature, growing in faith and love (Eph. 4:13-16).

Where does your team fall on the Healthy/Unhealthy scale?

HEALTHY							UNHEALTHY
Fullness	6	5	4	3	2	1	Emptiness
Hungry/Thirsty	6	5	4	3	2	1	Satisfied
Maturing	6	5	4	3	2	1	Immature
Formation	6	5	4	3	2	1	Information
Growth	6	5	4	3	2	1	Stagnation
Devotion	6	5	4	3	2	1	Busy-ness
Grounded	6	5	4	3	2	1	Tossed

____ Total Spiritual

Make some notes on your team's Spiritual Wellness here.

»   In what circumstances does your team exhibit Spiritual resilience?

»   What makes you feel vulnerable? What makes you hurt?

PART 2: LIFE IN COMMUNITY

Review the comments on Relational, Intellectual and Emotional brokenness and wellness in Lesson 7, "Ministry Threatens the Joy of Life in Community," and also the descriptions of biblical wellness given at the end of Lesson 7. 1.

What forces threatening your ministry team's Relational, Intellectual and Emotional Wellness resonate with you? How have you experienced that brokenness in your life together?

Relational Wellness

Rate each of the following:

Almost Never   **1**   **2**   **3**   **4**   **5**   **6**   *Almost Always*

____ The Spirit faithfully gives us the joy of showing patience toward others.

____ Our relationships reflect the Spirit's gift of unity, intrinsic to the body of Christ.

____ We are growing more humble, gentle, patient and loving (Eph. 4:2-6).

Where does your team fall on the Healthy/Unhealthy scale?

HEALTHY							**UNHEALTHY**
Respect	6	5	4	3	2	1	Contempt
Patience	6	5	4	3	2	1	Impatience
Loyalty	6	5	4	3	2	1	Treachery
Synergy	6	5	4	3	2	1	Division
Cleaving	6	5	4	3	2	1	Leaving
Servanthood	6	5	4	3	2	1	Selfishness
Trust	6	5	4	3	2	1	Suspicion

____ Total Relational

Make some notes on your team's Relational Wellness here.

» In what circumstances does your team exhibit Relational resilience?

» What makes you feel vulnerable? What makes you hurt?

Intellectual Wellness

Rate each of the following:

Almost Never   **1**   **2**   **3**   **4**   **5**   **6**   *Almost Always*

____ The Spirit faithfully gives us the joy of kindness and sincere listening.

____ We display a healthy curiosity about what we might learn from the wisdom of others.

____ We are learning to speak only truthful words that will build up those who hear (Eph. 4:25, 29).

Where does your team fall on the Healthy/Unhealthy scale?

HEALTHY							UNHEALTHY
Open	6	5	4	3	2	1	Closed
Honesty	6	5	4	3	2	1	Deception
Sharing	6	5	4	3	2	1	Hiding
Discovery	6	5	4	3	2	1	Ignorance
Curiosity	6	5	4	3	2	1	Prejudice
Compassion	6	5	4	3	2	1	Indifference
Listening	6	5	4	3	2	1	Attributing

____ Total Intellectual

Make some notes on your team's Intellectual Wellness here.

»   In what circumstances does your team exhibit Intellectual resilience?

»   What makes you feel vulnerable? What makes you hurt?

Emotional Wellbeing

Rate each of the following:

Almost Never   **1   2   3   4   5   6**   *Almost Always*

____ The Spirit faithfully gives us the joy of peace-filled relationships.

____ Our relationships in our work together are characterized by harmony.

____ We are growing in the graces of kindness, compassion and forgiveness (Eph. 4:26-32).

Where does your team fall on the Healthy/Unhealthy scale?

HEALTHY							UNHEALTHY
Sunny	6	5	4	3	2	1	Stormy
Light Mood	6	5	4	3	2	1	Dark Mood
Joyful	6	5	4	3	2	1	Serious
Harmony	6	5	4	3	2	1	Conflict
Grace	6	5	4	3	2	1	Grudges
Good Feelings	6	5	4	3	2	1	Hurt Feelings
Confession	6	5	4	3	2	1	Blame

___ Total Emotional

Make some notes on your team's Emotional Wellness here.

»   In what circumstances does your team exhibit Emotional resilience?

»   What makes you feel vulnerable? What makes you hurt?

PART 3: LIFE IN MINISTRY

Review the comments on Vocational, Physical and Financial brokenness and wellness in Lesson 8, "Ministry Threatens the Joy of Life in Ministry," and also the descriptions of biblical wellness given at the end of Lesson 8.1.

What forces threatening your ministry team's Vocational, Physical and Financial Wellness resonate with you? How have you experienced that brokenness in your life together?

Vocational Wellbeing

Rate each of the following:

Almost Never   **1**   **2**   **3**   **4**   **5**   **6**   *Almost Always*

____ The Spirit faithfully gives us the joy of serving others in a spirit of gentleness.

____ God's call to a life of service is an ever-increasing source of humility.

____ We are often able to recognize ways that God uses us to build up the body of Christ (Eph. 4:11-12).

Where does your team fall on the Healthy/Unhealthy scale?

HEALTHY							UNHEALTHY
Passion-driven	6	5	4	3	2	1	Job Description driven
Spirit-led	6	5	4	3	2	1	Ego-led
Joyful	6	5	4	3	2	1	Burdensome
Boundaries	6	5	4	3	2	1	Overfunctioning
Energized	6	5	4	3	2	1	Burnt out
Gitta	6	5	4	3	2	1	Gotta
Servant	6	5	4	3	2	1	Authority

____ Total Vocational

Make some notes on your team's Vocational Wellness here.

» In what circumstances does your team exhibit Vocational resilience?

» What makes you feel vulnerable? What makes you hurt?

Physical Wellbeing

Rate each of the following:

Almost Never   1   2   3   4   5   6   *Almost Always*

____ The Spirit faithfully gives us the joy of self-control as the flesh's passions are subdued.

____ Our physical health choices result in vitality for service to God, family and church.

____ While always present, our physical passions and desires do not control us (Eph. 4:17-20).

Where does your team fall on the Healthy/Unhealthy scale?

HEALTHY							UNHEALTHY
Rested	6	5	4	3	2	1	Exhausted
Eustress	6	5	4	3	2	1	Distress
Energy	6	5	4	3	2	1	Lethargy
Natural food	6	5	4	3	2	1	Processed food
Self-control	6	5	4	3	2	1	Lust
Active	6	5	4	3	2	1	Sedentary
Moderation	6	5	4	3	2	1	Indulgence

____ Total Physical

Make some notes on your team's Physical Wellness here.

» In what circumstances does your team exhibit Physical resilience?

» What makes you feel vulnerable? What makes you hurt?

Financial Wellbeing

Rate each of the following:

Almost Never   **1**   **2**   **3**   **4**   **5**   **6**   *Almost Always*

____ The Spirit faithfully gives us the joy of faithfulness in our stewardship of resources.

____ We respond appropriately to opportunities to show generosity.

____ We remember that we are provided for abundantly so we can share with those in need (Eph. 4:28).

Where does your team fall on the Healthy/Unhealthy scale?

HEALTHY							UNHEALTHY
Gratitude	6	5	4	3	2	1	Ingratitude
Sacrifice	6	5	4	3	2	1	Hoard
Contentment	6	5	4	3	2	1	Desire
Sharing	6	5	4	3	2	1	Accumulating
Planning	6	5	4	3	2	1	Chance
Trust	6	5	4	3	2	1	Fear
Generosity	6	5	4	3	2	1	Selfishness

____ Total Financial

Make some notes on your team's Financial Wellness here.

»   In what circumstances does your team exhibit Financial resilience?

»   What makes you feel vulnerable? What makes you hurt?

Where to Begin: Assessing Wellness

What does the above exercise indicate may be the aspect of your team's wellness from the Wellness Wheel that most needs the healing touch of Christ in your life together right now?

Do the assessment tools above match up with your own experience in recent months, affirming what you have sensed about your team's wellbeing?

If not, where do you feel you are currently experiencing the greatest need?

List here, in order of priority, which three aspects of wellness need your team's attention. We strongly encourage you to address the most critical need first, returning for work in the other areas only after you have experienced substantial healing in your first priority.

Our areas of growth:

Choose one for immediate attention:

Life with God   ____ Baptismal   ____ Spiritual

Life in Community   ____ Relational   ____ Intellectual ____ Emotional

Life in Ministry   ____ Vocational   ____ Physical   ____ Financial

Choose one for future consideration (after addressing the above):

Life with God   ____ Baptismal   ____ Spiritual

Life in Community   ____ Relational   ____ Intellectual ____ Emotional

Life in Ministry   ____ Vocational   ____ Physical   ____ Financial

Choose one for eventual consideration (after addressing both of the above):

Life with God   ____ Baptismal   ____ Spiritual

Life in Community   ____ Relational   ____ Intellectual ____ Emotional

Life in Ministry   ____ Vocational   ____ Physical   ____ Financial

LESSON TEN

Therefore, Self-Care Must Be Intentional

IT WOULD BE EASY TO SAY, "Elijah should have taken better care of himself!" It's hard to say exactly what he had been doing to care for his spiritual, emotional, relational and vocational wellbeing. 1 Kings 19 seems to indicate that he was in a significantly depleted condition. It makes us wonder how the story might have been different if Elijah had more fully tended to his own needs. We like to use the expression "self-care," but only under the broader umbrella of God's providential care for us. All of our care comes from our heavenly Father; he provides all we need to support this body and life. When we suggest that church workers be intentional about getting their own oxygen masks firmly in place before they tend to the needs of others, we're reminded that Someone else is providing the oxygen. The gift of bread and water that Elijah received from the hand of the Lord, as well as the gifts of rest, friends, and words of encouragement, all illustrate God's abiding, providing care for his children. God alone, through his Son Jesus Christ, is the fount of the daily healing that we need to continue on in ministry.

While only God can give us the healing we need, he's called us, just as he called Elijah, to exercise his gifts of wisdom and good judgment. Good daily and weekly disciplines will ensure our journey to the place where God can tend to our every need. The Lord does the healing; we go to the hospital. By grace, God restores us to the fullness of vitality and joy in ministry, and sends us back out the way we came to continue on until he decides that our work is done. It's in that sense that the wellness journey has led us to this final, concluding Lesson Ten to which we hope every church worker will finally arrive, "Self-care has to be intentional." Every wise disciple will make their own fitness for service a top priority and incorporate the daily habits of self-care into their lifestyle, the habits that invite the healing work of the Holy Spirit.[51]

We at Grace Place Wellness Ministries are not the first to suggest that called church workers put on their own oxygen masks before hustling to the aid of those traveling with them. Both of Paul's letters to Timothy do the same thing. In a word of encouragement that hints at the flight attendant's announcement on an airliner, Paul wrote, "You then, my son, be strong in the grace that is in Christ Jesus" (2 Timothy 2:1). The gifts of God are the only tools we have for ministry, and before administering the gifts of grace to the people of God, church workers must first be receivers. A better translation of the divine passive in this verse might say "be strengthened" in the grace of God. Paul is telling Timothy to remember first to safeguard his own wellbeing by drinking deeply of the refreshment and renewal that the Holy Spirit brings in the gospel of Christ's saving love.

Paul had future generations of church workers in mind when he continued, "And the things you have heard me say in the presence of many witnesses entrust to reliable men who will also be qualified to teach others" (2 Timothy 2:2). Did you notice the four generations of gospel proclamation, from Jesus to Paul, Paul to Timothy, then Timothy to others who will then pass it on to a fourth generation? Breathe in. "Be strengthened in grace." Breathe out. "Teach others." That's the pattern for wellness. Breathe in. Then breathe out. It's a pattern God set when he first breathed life into Adam and it still serves as our pattern for living and serving in ministry today. Lesson Ten could be summarized, "Don't forget to breathe!"

Over more than two decades, Grace Place Wellness Ministries has coached thousands of professional church workers and their spouses in the disciplines of Christian living for the sake of long, productive careers. Two assumptions undergird our ministry to ministers. Assumption 1: "I've been completely healed by the grace of God." Servants of Christ understand that because of salvation by grace through the finished work of the Savior, our work and deeds of ministry, no matter how glorious they may appear, contribute nothing to our life with God. Our humble works of service are nothing more than a response to God's healing in our lives, the natural outflow of God's saving grace found in the Spirit-led sanctified life. Assumption 2: "I'm in daily need of healing grace." Life in ministry is hard, and all of us are in continual need of the fortifying gifts of God to enable our continued faithful and fruitful work in the kingdom. While our redemption is full and complete, the wellness of church workers is a completely unfinished work. Every one of us is always only moments away from a traumatizing event that could potentially throw us under the broom tree. Our vitality for the work of ministry is daily diminished by the stress and strain of the tasks and is continually in need of refreshment. In the disciplines of daily renewal, we participate with God as we drink deeply of his good gifts.

Pastor and counselor David Ludwig, our retreat leader for many years, said it so well:

> Good self-care flows out of the new self that is a creation of God. Church leaders model what it means to value the gift of well-being. Sadly, many worn-out leaders model self-neglect rather than self-care. This is seen in patterns of overwork (doing "God's work"), isolation, neglect of health and fitness, imbalance of time and energy for family, self, God, and ministry. Ironically, attitudes that put self-care last and everything else first are symptoms of a ME-oriented focus ("It's all up to me").

When a leader takes care of self and strives for life balance, it reflects a WE-oriented awareness, because the person is more capable of service to the whole Body of Christ when in good health and experiencing well-being. As this internal struggle — ME vs. WE — is overcome by God's healing hand, self-aware adults take responsibility for creating a sense of well-being in their own body, mind and spirit — forming a healthy WE orientation within the self.[52]

Dr. Eckrich's vision for Grace Place Wellness Ministries has always been to offer wellness training for church workers, to inspire and equip them to care for their spiritual, relational, emotional and physical selves for the sake of the work of ministry. The first objective of our ministry was to stem the tide of church workers who were leaving the ministry far too soon. He also hoped to decrease the number of ministers who were removed from the ministry due to misbehavior, often the result of unmet personal needs that were not fulfilled in more appropriate ways.

Dr. Eckrich also sought to help congregations serve their function as the Lord's mission outposts for healing ministry in their communities by helping the leaders themselves experience the healing grace of Christ. By equipping ministry leaders with the passion and skills to seek out the healing grace of Christ in every dimension of their own lives, church workers become better able to lead their congregations to serve the hurting and broken so that they might also know the healing touch of Jesus. Breathe in, breathe out. First the minister is fed, and then the minister feeds. And when the congregation is well fed, they better serve their neighbors.

> **Breathe in, breathe out. First the minister is fed, and then the minister feeds.**

A third unexpected result of the ministry of Grace Place Wellness was the discovery that our work directly impacts the recruitment of young people into church work careers. The number of students at our church body's universities preparing for careers in church work is steadily declining. From time to time we have the opportunity to ask these students, "What concerns you most about a life in ministry?" For some reason, they are able to articulate, even before beginning their time of service, exactly the same stressors that we hear mentioned by experienced church workers on our retreats: unrealistic ministry expectations, neglect of family life, loneliness, and financial struggles. How would they possibly know that? These young people must be observing the church workers who serve them in their own home congregations, or, in the case of children of church workers, assessing the lifestyles of their parents. I intentionally ask church workers, "Which young people in your congregation want to be you when they grow up?" By helping church workers live healthy lives of joyful service, we're enhancing the recruitment efforts of the primary influencers of young people considering a life and career in Christian service: their own pastors, musicians and educators.

So what does a healthy church worker look like? The Barna report suggests that the common use of the term "robust," another word for "strong" to describe the preferred condition of healthy church workers, might be doing more harm than good. If we focus on raising up strong, "almost heroic" church workers, we're setting them up for failure. The report suggests instead a different image: resilience. "The pyramids of Giza are robust: big, impressive, immovable, unchangeable except by increments or an act of God. Yet given enough firepower, a single person could wipe them off the face of the earth. A forest, on the other hand, is resilient: at first glance, more vulnerable than the pyramids to a devastation-level event such as wildfire or attack by an invasive parasite. But wait a decade or a century, and the forest is likely to have recovered — and the soil beneath the trees to be richer, as well."[53] "Recovered" is a great way to put it. "Recovered" sounds a lot like the journey of Elijah. Resilient church workers are those that are sensitive to the unique hardships of this great calling, recognize when they have suffered spiritual, emotional, relational or vocational harm, and then utilize the resources that God gives for a time of recovery before launching back into their life callings. We learn to breathe in so we can breathe out again. Maybe that's one reason why so many of Jesus' parables were about fields and shrubs and living, growing things. Wellness in the kingdom of God is like the continuous cycle of growth; the seed falling to the ground, dying and rising again to bear fruit.

If a healthy professional church worker looks like a resilient forest, then what are the key characteristics of a church worker's intentional plan for recovery from the wounds of ministry and for the long-term disciplines of healthy, joyful living?

INTENTIONAL PLANS ARE GOSPEL-DRIVEN

I've been discouraged to discover that there's a reason why some church work professionals never learn the Ten Lessons on the journey to wellness. It may be that "Assumption #1" stated earlier in this chapter, that church workers are clear about the difference between justification and sanctification, is assuming too much, and you know what often results from assumptions. We've found over the years that a significant number of church workers are resistant to any conversation about self-care and the disciplines of Christian living because it smacks of legalism or pietism.

We're occasionally challenged by some who suggest that by encouraging intentional self-care, we're teaching a legalistic approach to Christian living. Our response, simply stated, is that at Grace Place Wellness we teach baptism. One of the things we love about The Wellness Wheel is the prominent way baptismal grace is positioned at the center hub of the wheel. The designers of the wheel, which included Dr. Eckrich, intentionally placed the phrase "In baptism – a new creation in Christ" at the nexus point for every other aspect of life. We begin all of our programs and retreats with a study of Baptismal Wellness. Every aspect of our life in Christ flows from and is enriched by the grace of God imparted in the Sacrament of Holy Baptism. Christian living is always grounded in the gifts granted in baptism.

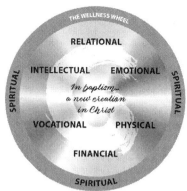

In his commentary on Colossians, Paul Deterding says it well: "Therefore, when the apostle exhorts his readers to put off the vices of the old man and to put on the virtues of the new man (Colossians 3:8, 12; see also Ephesians 4:22, 24), he is telling them to live the kind of life for which man was first created in God's image, which is the kind of life we will live when that image is fully restored in the new creation (Revelation 21-22). Having had the divine image restored to him in Baptism, the Christian is equipped to live that kind of life."[54] Is it possible for us to do that under our own strength and force of will? Not at all! "This putting off and putting on the Christian cannot do without continual reliance on God's grace in Christ and the aid of the Holy Spirit. Indeed, the Christian knows that any growth and improvement is not due to his own efforts, but is solely the result of the indwelling presence of Christ and his fruitful grace."[55] Christians are always learning to become what God has made them to be in their baptism, to learn to live the life that Christ is now living in him (see Galatians 2:20). That's the essence of Lesson Ten, to intentionally remember who you are and to drink deeply of God's gifts of grace.

> Christians are always learning to become what God has made them to be in their baptism.

An intentional plan for self-care is learning to put into daily practice the life of dying and rising, of putting off the old and putting on the new. As we learn to regularly, frequently reflect on our spiritual, relational, emotional and every other aspect of wellness, we're learning 1) to discern how the sinful nature has caused disruption and brokenness in that area of life; 2) to confess that sin, dying to the old nature and it's passions; 3) to be raised to new life by the promises of forgiveness and grace in the gospel; 4) to welcome the fruit of the Holy Spirit in his gifts of love, joy, peace, patience, kindness, goodness, faithfulness, gentleness and self-control; and then 5) to joyfully live obediently in the power of the gifts given, with joy, peace, patience, gentleness, etc. in the various vocations of life. These are the tools of intentionality that Paul encouraged Timothy to utilize.

The Formula of Concord teaches that,

> ...when people are born again through the Spirit of God and set free from the law (that is, liberated from its driving powers and driven by the Spirit of Christ), they live according to the unchanging will of God, as comprehended in the law, and do everything, insofar as they are reborn, from a free and merry spirit. Works of this kind are not, properly speaking, works of the law but works and fruits of the Spirit, or, as Paul calls them, 'the law of the mind' and 'the law of Christ.' For such people are 'no longer under law but under grace,' as St. Paul says in Romans 8. [Rom 7:23; 6:14] [56]

In this life believers are able to live "from a free and merry spirit" only imperfectly. We're learning as we go, but each day is a new beginning.

DESIGNING AN INTENTIONAL WELLNESS PLAN

It's time to get started on the challenging work of designing and implementing an intentional plan for your wellness. Growth as a disciple of Christ and a servant of the gospel means continually learning from the experiences of life so far. A wellness plan will help you to incorporate the wisdom you have gained along the way, those practices that fill and restore you, that keep you resilient and healthy as you face the trails of life. More importantly, designing a wellness plan will help you discern the unwise behaviors that have led to a diminished capacity for healthy living. You'll be asking questions about your Life with God, your Life in Community with family, friends, co-workers and the people your serve, and your Life in Ministry. You'll consider what are you doing that you should not be doing because it's detrimental to your wellbeing. You'll also consider what disciplines you are not practicing that might enhance your resilience, your response-ability, your vitality and ultimately your joy in ministry.

Hopefully, as you've worked your way through the Ten Lessons on the journey to wellness, you've been evaluating your own practices of self-care. I expect you've noted those practices that have been helpful in the past and considering some new ones that you can incorporate into your daily life. I hope also that you've begun to identify that particular aspect of life, whether spiritual, emotional, vocational, relational or physical that needs the Lord's healing touch and your special attention as you move forward in wellness. You might have some ideas in mind for implementation right away. That's the work of God the Holy Spirit, imparting his wisdom. That's reason to be thankful!

Before you begin developing your plan, I want to encourage you to take a look at the Appendix following this chapter where we'll introduce you to a resource developed to guide you in your discernment process. The Reclaiming the Joy of Ministry Workbook Series outlines a step-by-step process to help you develop the plan that fits your own history, temperament and current needs. Learn more about the Workbook Series at **GracePlaceWellness.org**.

If you feel ready to design a wellness plan of your own, I'd encourage you to incorporate the following qualities that we utilize in the Workbook Series.

INTENTIONAL WELLNESS PLANS ARE COMPREHENSIVE

The Wellness Wheel is by no means inspired, but we find it an appropriately comprehensive enough model for our purposes for a number of reasons. The eight aspects of wellness that are identified on the Wheel are far-reaching enough to address just about every issue of Christian living that church workers, (or any disciples of Christ), are likely to face in the course of any season of life. We also appreciate how The Wellness Wheel lends itself nicely to the three sub-categories we've previously mentioned: Life with God, Life in Community and Life in Ministry.

INTENTIONAL WELLNESS PLANS ARE REALISTIC

How many heroes are there in the Bible? The answer, of course, is that there is only one Hero in the Bible. The rest of the characters are just sinner/saints who, by the grace of God, were called, healed, filled, sent and blessed for service in the kingdom. When Christian ministry is fruitful, it's because the Hero has been at work through our humble, imperfect acts of service. Elijah is an excellent example of the spiritual, physical, emotional and vocational frailties of the humans that God calls into his service. It's no mistake that the inspired Word of the Lord includes this episode from Elijah's life that shows a giant of the faith at his very worst. The beauty of the Bible is that it is, first and foremost, grounded in real history and in the lives of real people just like you and me, Elijah and Peter, and hundreds of others. It's our story and it's real life. An intentional plan addresses the real challenges of ministry in the places where it really hurts.

INTENTIONAL WELLNESS PLANS ARE BIBLICAL

God's mending and restorative/redemptive work is on display throughout the course of the biblical narrative, from Genesis to Revelation. An intentional plan will examine the whole Bible's encouragement, instruction, correction and grace for living.

In our programming, we've found that Ephesians 4 serves as a simple summary outline of the scriptural teaching on wellness. Each of the eight aspects of life identified in The Wellness Wheel are mentioned, and while not exhaustive, Ephesians 4 is inclusive. We also like to emphasize Paul's encouragement for life by the Spirit in Galatians 5, specifically verses 22-24 where he delineates the power of Christian living found in Christ's continuing work in his people, the fruit of the Spirit. As a guide and as a simple, but not simplistic handle on The Wellness Wheel, we like to connect each of the eight aspects of wellness with one of the facets of the Spirit's fruit described in Galatians 5, the Spirit's gift of joy being the overarching indicator of church worker wellbeing.

INTENTIONAL WELLNESS PLANS ARE MISSIONAL

Church worker wellness is not "self-help." If you want a life of sunshine and lollipops, you're in the wrong business. St. Paul even suggested that he'd be better off dead than continuing in his mission work: "I desire to depart and be with Christ, which is better by far; but it is more necessary for you that I remain in the body" (Philippians 1:23-24). Our desire, and we believe the desire of Jesus, is for you to be healthy, resilient and invigorated as you remain in the body for a little while longer, not for your own pleasure and benefit, but for the sake of the work of ministry to which you've been called. That's what makes an intentional design for self-care critically important for all church workers. Ministers of the gospel take responsibility for their own response-ability. By tending to your own spiritual, emotional, relational, financial and physical needs, you'll be, to the best of the capacity that God in his wisdom allows, ready to respond to his call to service in the kingdom and to the needs of those who need help getting their own oxygen masks in place.

INTENTIONAL WELLNESS PLANS ARE SIMPLE

Because life in church and school ministry is rarely what you would call easy, you'll want to do your best to keep the journey to wellness as simple as possible. We encourage you to find a meaningful scripture passage, like Ephesians 4, as a guiding text and to use the fruit of the Spirit as markers of wellness to keep your plan for healing and growth simple and useful. Simple, easy to remember handles on wellness are easier to access in moments of stress and anxiety when you need an immediate assessment of wellness to help you take the beginning steps to getting back on track quickly.

INTENTIONAL WELLNESS PLANS ARE PERSONAL

An intentional plan requires you to do some significant reflection on your past: Where has the Lord been leading you so far? What digressions along the way are in need of confession and forgiveness? Where have you been resistant to change? You'll need to envision your healthier future. Who do you trust to offer wisdom, counsel and encouragement along the way? Are there disciplines of the faith with which you are not familiar, but that you feel compelled to try? What do you teach others about this aspect of wellness in their lives that you could apply to your own? The intentional growth plan that you put together for your own self-care needs to be the most personalized one possible, one that only you can design.

INTENTIONAL WELLNESS PLANS ARE CONGREGATIONAL

Since the very beginning of the Christian church, leaders in the church have recognized the symbiotic relationship that exists between congregations and their leaders. Back in Lesson Four, "Don't try this alone," we looked at Paul's longing for mutual blessing with the Romans: "I long to see you so that I may impart to you some spiritual gift to make you strong, that is, that you and I may be mutually encouraged by each other's faith" (Romans 1:11-12).

The close connection between congregational health and church worker health will be a significant portion of the wellness plan that you develop. The body of Christ and all of its members work and serve and learn and grow together. Healthy members make healthy congregations and healthy congregations make healthy members.

A brief pamphlet called, "Healthy Congregations. Healthy Leaders" introduced The Wellness Wheel back in 1997, and concluded with these words for church leaders.

> The heartbreaking experience of pastoral crisis that the Apostle Paul described in the first century does not have to be the norm for congregations today. It is possible for congregations to be intentional about making themselves hospitable environments for the flourishing of ministry and ministers. To do this, congregations need to look at all of the dimensions of ministerial life and ask if the conditions are what they should be. Is the congregation encouraging the physical, social, emotional, vocational, intellectual, economic, and spiritual life of its ministers? The answer comes when intentional work is done in all areas.[57]

It's that intentional work that we hope you and those you serve will engage in together.

If you serve in a context that provides a healthy setting for church workers and their families, you've been given a great gift. They will be a tremendous support for you as you continue on the wellness journey outlined in the next section. If your context is less than healthy, please find encouragement from knowing that your loving Father in heaven wants the very best for you and for those you serve, and your journey to wellness can be the very first part of your church's journey also.

NOT FINISHED YET!

» Take a few minutes to consider whether Lesson Ten, "Self-care has to be intentional" is a lesson about ministry that you've taken to heart.

» What did you read in this chapter that resonates most deeply? What made you say to yourself, "That's really true!"?

» How would you phrase Lesson Ten differently?

» What did Darrell not discuss in this chapter that really could have been mentioned?

» If this is a lesson you've already learned from your own experience, when did you first discover that it was true?

» What needs your further contemplation before moving on to the next chapter?

MINISTRY TEAM CONVERSATION STARTERS FOR LESSON TEN

» What would be different if your ministry team were more intentional about your Life with God (Baptismal and Spiritual Wellness)?

» How might it help you flourish in your ministry?

» What would be different if your ministry team were more intentional about your Life in Community (Relational, Intellectual, and Emotional Wellness)?

» How might it help you flourish in your ministry?

» What would be different if your ministry team were more intentional about your Life in Ministry (Vocational, Physical, and Financial Wellness)?

» How might it help you flourish in your ministry?

» Who will be responsible for your team's intentional wellness plan?

» How will you address together the areas for growth that you identified at the end of Lesson Nine?

Appendix

RECLAIMING THE JOY OF MINISTRY WORKBOOK SERIES

The *Reclaiming the Joy of Ministry* Workbook Series is a simple, self-directed Discovery Guide, grounded in the study of scripture, that is designed to help you ask hard questions about yourself and seek answers from the Lord who heals and restores joy. Wellness is not perfection, but it is experiencing the healing touch of Christ where you need it; in your Life with God, Your Life in Community or in your Life in Ministry. The Workbook Series is the fruit of our more than twenty years of experience leading professional church workers and their spouses to rediscover the joy of ministry by renewal, refreshment, and re-creation in the gospel of Jesus Christ. Get more information on the Workbook Series at **GracePlaceWellness.org**.

THE MISSION OF GRACE PLACE WELLNESS MINISTRIES

Grace Place Wellness nurtures vitality and joy in ministry
*by **inspiring and equipping** church workers to lead healthy lives.*

The Ten Lessons covered in *Reclaiming the Joy of Ministry* have been intentionally designed to be ***inspiring***, with the hope that those who study the Lessons will learn better how to "***lead healthy lives***," seeking wholeness in every aspect of life. In the Workbooks, our ministry of equipping is presented in a step-by-step, self-directed study culminating in a biblically based, gospel-centered guide for wellness, just as thousands have developed at our week-long retreats and wellness conferences around the world.

Healing is never a work we do in ourselves. The Workbook Series is not a self-help plan, but truly a journey to that "Place of Grace" under the care of a loving God who, as long as he chooses to wake you each morning, has plans for you in his kingdom's work! A personal wellness plan that really works must be a plan of your own design. Only you know the hurts and the brokenness that you have experienced along the way, so only you, with the Holy Spirit's guiding and care, can discover the path back to wellness. Your journey will be unique. We believe that just as God knew what Elijah needed on the mountaintop retreat, he knows exactly what you need to rediscover the joy that fuels ministry or to keep that joy alive. We want to help you find the Lord's next steps for your adventure of faith and service!

KEY COMPONENTS OF THE *RECLAIMING THE JOY OF MINSTRY* WORKBOOK SERIES

In brief outline, the model is built around these simple components that were first presented following Lessons Six, Seven and Eight:

	The Wellness Wheel	The JOY of...	The Fruit of the Spirit Is...	Ephesians Four "A life worthy of the calling..."
My Life with God	Baptismal	Identity	Love	Ephesians 4:21-24
	Spiritual	Receptivity	Goodness	Ephesians 4:13-16
My Life in Community	Relational	Unity	Patience	Ephesians 4:2-6
	Intellectual	Curiosity	Kindness	Ephesians 4:25, 29
	Emotional	Harmony	Peace	Ephesians 4:26, 30-32
My Life in Ministry	Vocational	Humility	Gentleness	Ephesians 4:11-12
	Physical	Vitality	Self-Control	Ephesians 4:17-20
	Financial	Generosity	Faithfulness	Ephesians 4:28

Appendix

USING MY WELLNESS JOURNEY

Wellness, like discipleship, is a journey, not a destination. The process that you will encounter in each section of The Workbook Series is designed to lead you on your own personal journey from your current situation to a new, more vibrant and more joyful state by welcoming the healing touch of God the Holy Spirit. It's a plan for developing a preventive wellness strategy to keep you at your best for a long, healthy career in ministry.

A discovery process takes time. As the Lord works in you through his Word of law, (indicating unhealthy choices and creating dissatisfaction with your current state), and as he works in you through his Word of gospel, (granting healing, peace, restoration and the return of joy), you will experience numerous times of both frustration and gladness, of confession and forgiveness, of struggle and celebration. That's the way it has always been for those whom their loving Father is teaching and disciplining. The important thing is to get started.

There are eight Discovery Guides, one corresponding to each of the eight aspects of wellness outlined in The Wellness Wheel: Baptismal, Spiritual, Relational, Intellectual, Emotional, Vocational, Physical and Financial. Each individual Discovery Guide is broken down into four separate sections, each section building on the work of the preceding, culminating in your personally designed plan to welcome Christ's healing touch. We recommend working on just one aspect of wellness at a time, beginning with your most critical need as you began to identify in the assessment at the conclusion of Lesson Nine.

Each of the eight Discovery Guides follows the same five part outline.

STEP ONE: UNDERSTANDING WELLNESS

In Step One you will be introduced to some of the key elements of the aspect of wellness you are addressing. You'll be invited to study and reflect on the nature of wellness as depicted in the scriptures for any of the eight aspects of wellness outlined on the Wellness Wheel. You will be encouraged to consider a simple Marker of Wellbeing we have used to guide others as you examine your own walk by the fruit of the Spirit as it relates to your life. In particular, you'll be asked to identify the sources of joy that you experience in this aspect of your walk with God and your walk with others. At the completion of this Step, you will have developed your own understanding of the aspect of wellness chosen for your attention developed through your reflections on each of the following. (The Markers of Wellness and One Word Definitions are those outlined at the end of Chapters Six, Seven and Eight.) The process asks you to consider...

- ▸ A One Word Definition of Wellness (see chart above)

- ▸ A Reflection on the Marker of Wellness

- ▸ A Bible Study on The Fruit of the Spirit (see chart above)

- ▸ Experiencing the Joy of Wellness

- ▸ Devotional Resources on Your Journey

- ▸ A Summary Conclusion of Step One: My Understanding of the Scripture's Teaching on Wellness

STEP TWO: UNDERSTANDING BROKENNESS

In Step Two you'll be challenged to consider what has become broken in your life. Why has this aspect of wellness become that part of your journey that is in need of the Lord's gracious, healing touch? What forces around you and which choices that you've made have contributed to the depletion of your joy and the discomfort you're currently enduring? You'll be asked to define your current reality by clearly articulating what's going on in your heart, your mind and your spirit. This will prepare you to seek the renewal that God is always ready to offer his children. At the completion of this Step, you will have outlined your own brokenness according to the experiences you have endured and your response to those experiences. The process asks you to consider...

- ▶ The Way of the Cross

- ▶ A Review of My Self-Assessment

- ▶ Some Indicators of Brokenness in Church Workers

- ▶ Determining the Causes of My Own Brokenness

- ▶ Assessing My Self-Awareness

- ▶ Examples of Others Experiencing Similar Brokenness

- ▶ A Summary Conclusion of Step Two: How Am I Experiencing Brokenness?

STEP THREE: UNDERSTANDING HEALING

Step Three will help you to envision the desired future condition you seek, by the grace of God through his healing care. Through consideration of biblical examples and remembering your own personal history of blessing under God's providential care, you will start to define what wellness might look like for you. You'll also begin to count the costs involved in making new choices that will open you to new beginnings, putting off the old nature, being made new in Christ, and putting on the new nature to walk by the Spirit (Ephesians Four:Two1-TwoFour), renewed and refreshed for days ahead. At the completion of this Step, you will have gained a clearer understanding of what (Spiritual, Emotional, Relational, Physical, etc.) wellness would look like in your own situation after having welcomed the healing work of the gospel into your life. The process asks you to consider...

- A Study of Ephesians Four

- Examining My Past History of Wellness

- Anticipating the Experience of Christ's Healing Touch

- A Study of the Spirit's Work of Substantial Healing

- Identifying Gospel Resources for Renewal

- Suggested Reading

- Identifying Congregational, Denominational and Community Resources

- Identifying Coaching, Mentoring, Counseling or Spiritual Direction Assistance

- A Summary Conclusion of Step Three: My Vision for (Spiritual, Emotional, etc.) Wellness

STEP FOUR: WELCOMING THE HEALING SPIRIT

In Step Four you will be guided through a planning process to help you begin to eliminate or at least better manage the forces that are contributing to your brokenness and to find the healing care that God provides in the gospel resources of Word and Sacrament and in your communities of care and encouragement. Before you begin Step Four, you'll be asked to consider whether or not it is necessary to seek healing for past wounds before making plans for the future in Step Five. At the completion of this Step, should you choose to work through the healing process, you will have developed a specific, measurable self-care action plan for putting the past behind. The process asks you to consider...

- Drafting a Goal Statement for Restorative Care

- Developing a Gospel-Centered Action Plan

- Monitoring the Journey and Outlining Accountability and Encouragement

- A Summary Conclusion of Step Four: An Action Plan for Restorative Care

STEP FIVE: WELCOMING THE SPIRIT OF JOY

In Step Five you will be guided through a planning process to help you begin to chart a plan for the long-term journey of wellness, breaking habits of the past that have led to anxiety and distress and establishing new patterns of behavior that will contribute to establishment of boundaries and increased vitality and joy in ministry. You'll consider what resources of nurture and blessing you will need along the journey as you walk by faith, never perfectly healed, but bound and fortified for the next phase of faithfulness in your calling. At the completion of this Step, you will have developed a specific, measurable self-care action plan for your chosen aspect of wellness. The process asks you to consider...

- Drafting a Goal Statement for (Spiritual, Relational, Vocational, etc.) Wellness

- Developing a Gospel-Centered Action Plan

- Monitoring the Journey and Outlining Accountability and Encouragement

- A Summary Conclusion of Step Four: An Action Plan for Vitality and Joy

A FINAL WORD OF ENCOURAGEMENT

Elijah's journey from Mount Carmel to Mount Horeb was a long one, and the journey back to joy in ministry didn't come easy, but when he was in desperate need of the healing touch of the Lord he took the first step and went to the mountain, and our loving God brought him back to the place of wholeness. You might be on a ministry mountaintop right now. I hope and pray that you are. But whether you're on a mountaintop, in a deep valley or riding the roller coaster in between, you need an intentional, gospel-focused wellness plan of your own, because ministry, always great, is getting harder and harder. We'd love to be your companion along the way. Thousands and thousands of your fellow servants of the gospel, dating all the way back to Elijah, have found refreshment and renewal from a God who binds up the wounded and sends them back into joyful service once again. I know that he has plans for you, too.

I'd like to conclude with a word of encouragement from Dr. Luther that we began with.

> The new leaven is the faith and grace of the Spirit. It does not leaven the whole lump at once, but gently, and gradually, we become like this new leaven and eventually, a bread of God. This life, therefore, is not godliness but the process of becoming godly, not health but getting well, not being but becoming, not rest but exercise. We are not now what we shall be, but we are on the way. The process is not yet finished, but it is actively going on. This is not the goal but it is the right road. At present, everything does not gleam and sparkle, but everything is being cleansed.[58]

God bless you with joy in ministry as you walk by faith under his abiding care!

Endnotes

Introduction

1   Dr. Eckrich eventually left his medical practice to lead Grace Place Wellness Ministries fulltime.

2   Martin Luther, *Defense and Explanation of All the Articles*, Luther's Works: American Edition, Vol. 32, (Philadelphia: Fortress, 1958), p. 24.

Lesson 1

3   The following discussion is informed by Walter A. Maier III, "1 Kings 12-22", Concordia Commentary (St Louis: 2019) pp. 1404-1438.

Lesson 2

4   C. F. W. Walther, *The Proper Distinction between Law and Gospel*, trans. W. H. T. Dau, (St. Louis: Concordia Publishing House, 1928), p. 285.

5   Ibid.

6   *Lutheran Service Book*, "Collect For Guidance in our Calling," (St Louis: Concordia Publishing House, 2006), p. 311.

Lesson 3

7   Maier, 1 Kings 12-22, p. 1429, author's emphasis.

8   www.lcms.org/about/seven-mission-priorities

9   https://wellbeing.nd.edu/assets/198819/emerging_insights_2_1_.pdf

10   Ibid, p. 10.

11   Ibid, p. 21.

12   Ibid, p. 11

13 Susan Howatch wrote a series of novels known as The Starbridge Series, beginning with "Glittering Images," (Ballantine, 1987). The novels wind their way through most of the early twentieth century following the often intertwining lives of generations of clergy, from parish pastors to Anglican bishops, and the way they and their families respond to the pressures and challenges of life in ministry. The core issue for most of the central characters is the matter of image versus reality. "What would people think if they really knew me?" Much of the time, the protagonist in the story doesn't even know himself. They've often bought into their own "glittering image."

14 Paul David Tripp, *Dangerous Calling: Confronting the Unique Challenges of Pastoral Ministry*, (Wheaton, IL: Crossway Publishers, 2012), p. 33.

15 *The Green Lantern*. Directed by Martin Campbell, (Los Angeles: Warner Bros., DeLine Pictures, 2011.

16 Gary L. Harbaugh, *Pastor as Person: Maintaining Personal Integrity in the Choices and Challenges of Ministry*, (Minneapolis: Augsburg, 1984) p. 60, author's emphasis).

Lesson 4

17 Rev. Doug Dommer, Salem Lutheran Church, Tomball, TX in his farewell sermon after 38 years, 3/31/19.

Lesson 5

18 Frederick Buechner, *Listening to Your Life: Daily Meditations with Frederick Buechner*, (New York: HarperCollins, 1992), pp. 286-7. Originally published in The Hungering Dark.

19 Buechner, *Listening to Your Life*, pp. 287-288.

20 John Piper, **www.desiringgod.org/articles/how-do-you-define-joy** July 25, 2015.

21 *The Book of Concord: The Confessions of the Evangelical Lutheran Church*, Edited by Robert Kolb and Timothy J. Wengert, Translated by Charles Arand, et. al. (Minneapolis: Fortress Press, 2000). Small Catechism, p. 360.

22 Ibid.

23 Matthew Harrison, "Joyfully Lutheran: Report to the District Conventions", (LCMS Office of the President, 2018).

Lesson 6

24 Garth D. Ludwig, *Order Restored: A Biblical Interpretation of Health, Medicine and Healing*, (St. Louis: Concordia Publishing House, 1999), p 27.

25 Originally labelled "The Lutheran Wellness Wheel," it was developed by the Inter-Lutheran Coordinating Council on Ministerial Health and Wellness in 2009. Dr. John Eckrich, the founder of Grace Place Wellness Ministries, was among those consulting in the development of The Wellness Wheel. The model has served our ministry well

Endnotes

as a basic paradigm for all of our wellness programming. Many organizations use a wellness wheel to illustrate the multi-faceted character of human life, some with as few as four or five segments, others with as many as eighteen or twenty.

26 Others who use The Lutheran Wellness Wheel as their guiding paradigm usually speak of only seven aspects of wellness and do not include baptism into Christ (in the center of the wheel) as a separate category. Their thought is that baptism touches every other aspect of life, but is not a category in itself. In our teaching model, we've found the topic of baptismal living to be both distinctive on its own as a category of wellness and also foundational for understanding all the others.

27 John W. Kleinig, *Grace upon Grace: Spirituality for Today*, (St. Louis: Concordia Publishing House, 2008), p. 12.

28 Barna, p. 20.

29 Ibid.

30 *The Book of Concord*, Large Catechism, p. 400.

31 *Children's Letters to God: The New Collection*, Compiled by Stuart Hample and Eric Marshall, (New York: Workman Publishing, 1991), p. 25.

32 Wesley, sermon dated December 1, 2019. **https://www.washingtonpost.com/religion/2019/12/11/i-feel-so-distant-god-popular-dc-area-pastor-confesses-hes-tired-announces-sabbatical**

Lesson 7

33 *Lutheran Service Book*, (St Louis: Concordia Publishing House, 2006), p. 644, stz. 2.

34 Bob Burns, Tasha D. Chapman, Donald Guthrie, *Resilient in Ministry: What Pastors Told Us about Surviving and Thriving*, (Downers Grove, IL: InterVarsity Press, 2013), p. 170.

35 Barna, p. 38.

36 Ibid., p. 40.

Lesson 8

37 Walther, *Law and Gospel*, p. 285.

38 *The Book of Concord*, Small Catechism, p. 354.

39 The Duke University Clergy Health Initiative has studied clergy wellbeing extensively for the past generation. The lead researchers have produced an excellent overview of their findings in *Fractured and Faithful: Responding to the Clergy Health Crisis*, by Rae Jean Proeschold-Bell and Jason Byassee, (Grand Rapids: Baker, 2018). See also **www.clergyhealthinitiative.org**

40 Thom S. Rainer, **www.ThomRainer.com** Blog 11/12/18

Lesson 9

41 *Theological Dictionary of the New Testament*, Vol. VII, p. 990.

42 See also Psalm 30:2, Jeremiah 17:14, Hosea 6:1, Jeremiah 30:17, Psalm 103:3, etc.

43 The bronze serpent on a pole later became the symbol of the healing arts known as the caduceus.

44 Henri J.M. Nouwen, *The Wounded Healer: Ministry in Contemporary Society*, (New York: Doubleday Image, 1990), p. 72.

45 Walther, *Law and Gospel*, p. 23.

46 Francis Schaeffer, *True Spirituality*, (Wheaton, IL: Tyndale House Publishers, 1971), p. 179-180.

47 Ibid., p. 132.

48 Luther's Small Catechism, Explanation of the First Article of the Apostles' Creed.

49 Luther's Small Catechism, Explanation of the Second Article of the Apostles' Creed.

50 Luther's Small Catechism, Explanation of the Third Article of the Apostles' Creed.

Lesson 10

51 Dr. Leopoldo Sánchez has provided excellent guidance on the Holy Spirit's work of shaping, forming and healing his children in *Sculptor Spirit: Models of Sanctification from Spirit Christology*, (Downers Grove, IL: IVP Academic, 2019). We strongly encourage attention to this Christ-centered, biblical model when developing an intentional plan for seeking the Spirit's healing gifts.

52 David J. Ludwig, Mary R. Jacobs, *Christian Concepts for Care: Understanding and Helping People with Mental Health Issues*, (St. Louis: Concordia Publishing House, 2014), p. 138.

53 Barna, p. 155, first cited by Stanley McCrystal in "Team of Teams."

54 Paul E. Deterding, *Colossians*, (St Louis: Concordia Publishing House, 2003), p. 151.

55 Ibid., p. 155. See also Deterding's description of Christ as "the epitome, enabler and example of the Christian life," p. 159.

56 *The Book of Concord*, Formula of Concord/Solid Declaration, p. 590. See also, Large Catechism, Creed, 69 (Kolb, p. 440); Apology of the Augsburg Confession, XV, 45-47 (Kolb, pp. 229-230); Formula of Concord/Epitome, II, 17 (Kolb, p. 494); Large Catechism, Preface, 20 (Kolb, p. 383).

57 James P. Wind, *Healthy Congregations, Healthy Leaders*, (St. Louis: LCMS Ministerial Growth and Support, 2009), p. 30.

Appendix

58 *Luther's Works*, vol. 32, p. 24.

Made in the USA
Columbia, SC
15 March 2022